Women's Health
in Mainland Southeast Asia

Women's Health in Mainland Southeast Asia has been co-published simultaneously as *Women & Health*, Volume 35, Number 4 2002.

Women's Health in Mainland Southeast Asia

Andrea Whittaker, PhD
Editor

Women's Health in Mainland Southeast Asia has been co-published simultaneously as *Women & Health*, Volume 35, Number 4 2002.

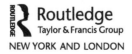

Routledge
Taylor & Francis Group
NEW YORK AND LONDON

First published by
The Haworth Press, Inc.
10 Alice Street
Binghamton, N Y 13904-1580

This edition published 2011 by Routledge

Routledge   Routledge
Taylor & Francis Group   Taylor & Francis Group
711 Third Avenue   2 Park Square, Milton Park
New York, NY 10017   Abingdon, Oxon OX14 4RN

Women's Health in Mainland Southeast Asia has been co-published simultaneously as *Women & Health*, Volume 35, Number 4 2002.

The development, preparation, and publication of this work has been undertaken with great care. However, the publisher, employees, editors, and agents of The Haworth Press and all imprints of The Haworth Press, Inc., including The Haworth Medical Press® and Pharmaceutical Products Press®, are not responsible for any errors contained herein or for consequences that may ensue from use of materials or information contained in this work. Opinions expressed by the author(s) are not necessarily those of The Haworth Press, Inc. With regard to case studies, identities and circumstances of individuals discussed herein have been changed to protect confidentiality. Any resemblance to actual persons, living or dead, is entirely coincidental.

Cover design by Jennifer M. Gaska
Cover photography by Maxine Whittaker
The textile/fabric on the cover, courtesy of the editor, Andrea Whittaker

Library of Congress Cataloging-in-Publication Data

Women's health in mainland Southeast Asia / Andrea Whittaker, editor.
    p. ; cm. – (Women & health ; v. 35, no. 4)
    Includes bibliographical references and index.
    ISBN 0-7890-1988-4 (hard : alk. paper)–ISBN 0-7890-1989-2 (pbk : alk. paper)
    1. Women–Asia, Southeastern–Health and hygiene. 2. Women's health services–Asia, Southeastern.
    [DNLM: 1. Women's Health–Asia, Southeastern. 2. Health Services Accessibility–Asia, Southeastern. 3. Socioeconomic Factors–Asia, Southeastern. 4. Women, Working–Asia, Southeastern. WA 309 W8734 2002] I. Whittaker, Andrea (Andrea N.) II. Series.
RA541.A785 .W664 2002
362.1′082′0959–dc21

                                             2002006958

Women's Health in Mainland Southeast Asia

CONTENTS

ABOUT THE EDITOR

Andrea Whittaker, PhD, is Joint Lecturer at the Key Center for Women's Health in Society and the Melbourne Institute of Asian Languages and Societies, University of Melbourne. She is a medical anthropologist whose primary research interests and publications relate to women's health, reproductive health, and gender and primary health care in Thailand and Australia. Dr. Whittaker's most recent book, *Intimate Knowledge: Women and Their Health in North-East Thailand* (2000) is an ethnography of women's health practices in a rural Thai village. She is currently completing a major project on illegal abortion in Thailand.

Introduction:
Reflections on Gender, Power and Health in Mainland Southeast Asia

Andrea Whittaker, PhD

Dramatic changes have marked the past few decades in mainland Southeast Asia. Thailand has experienced rapid economic boom and bust, industrialization and increasing urbanization. Vietnam and Laos are managing a transition from centrally planned economies to increased liberalization with concurrent social transformation. Cambodia struggles to maintain peace and emerge from years of war. Burma has been internationally isolated since the imposition of the current military regime.

The picture of health status in these countries remains diverse. Thailand's health profile reflects its economic development and the concomitant expansion of health services throughout the country. Basic primary health care programs promoting maternal and child health, immunization, water and sanitation have decreased mortality from major infectious diseases, pregnancy and childbirth in most regions of the

Andrea Whittaker is Joint Lecturer, Key Center for Women's Health in Society, and the Melbourne Institute of Asian Languages and Societies, The University of Melbourne, Melbourne, Victoria, 3010, Australia (E-mail: a.whittaker@unimelb.edu.au).

The author wishes to thank Eloise Brown of the University of Melbourne for her assistance in preparing the manuscripts of this collection and Lenore Manderson for her editorial suggestions. The author also wishes to thank the anonymous reviewers for their comments.

[Haworth co-indexing entry note]: "Introduction: Reflections on Gender, Power and Health in Mainland Southeast Asia." Whittaker, Andrea. Co-published simultaneously in *Women & Health* (The Haworth Medical Press, an imprint of The Haworth Press, Inc.) Vol. 35, No. 4, 2002, pp. 1-6; and: *Women's Health in Mainland Southeast Asia* (ed: Andrea Whittaker) The Haworth Medical Press, an imprint of The Haworth Press, Inc., 2002, pp. 1-6. Single or multiple copies of this article are available for a fee from The Haworth Document Delivery Service [1-800-HAWORTH, 9:00 a.m. - 5:00 p.m. (EST). E-mail address: getinfo@haworthpressinc.com].

country. In addition, a successful family planning program has contributed to a lowering of fertility. The overall trend in Thailand is the increased prevalence of 'lifestyle diseases' such as cardiovascular diseases and neoplasms. Other countries in the region have less primary health care infrastructure and fewer resources. This is reflected in health indicators showing poor maternal and infant mortality rates and high fertility and a high incidence of morbidity and mortality from preventable diseases, nutritional deficiencies, malaria and parasitic infections.

Despite the differences, all countries are now confronted with the AIDS pandemic. As in other parts of the world, AIDS exposes the discrepancies between rich and poor countries in their ability and willingness to respond. While Thailand has had considerable success in developing a prevention program, it struggles to provide services to the increasing number of people living with HIV. Other countries in the region still grapple to implement prevention strategies.

This collection focuses upon the ways in which women's health is situated within the social, cultural, and economic context of the region. The six papers are based upon research in Vietnam, Cambodia, Burma, and Thailand, from a range of perspectives. All the papers are based upon ethnographic research and attempt to convey something of the lived experiences of women. All move beyond the simple stereotypical equation of woman's health as maternal and child health. All engage with the broader context of social change and its effects upon health. In doing so, they explore two major themes: the political economy of health reflected through the inter-relationship between women's health, work and social position, and the social meanings of women's bodies and health. They draw attention to gendered power relations that directly and indirectly impinge upon women's health status.

The first two papers focus upon women as workers. Sally Theobald's paper situates health within the broader context of women's lives and the conditions of their changing economic roles. Industrialization has both provided new opportunities for women as migrant workers, and new dangers to their health. Theobald's paper gives an account of the gendered structures and organization of work in electronics factories in Northern Thailand. The women in these factories suffer from a range of health problems, from work-related stress to chemical hazards. Her analysis traces the distribution of risks along gendered lines, and the reasons why women continue to work in these environments despite their knowledge of the dangers. As she notes, the health effects from working in this industry extend beyond the factory gates, to high-risk behaviors, such as the regular use of stimulants, analgesics, alcohol abuse, drunk-driving and driving while fatigued. Casual sex, unplanned pregnancies and STDs are double-edged–they constitute major risks for women but also allow for accusations and rumors that women factory workers who claim work-related chemical poisoning are, in fact, all suffering the effects of HIV/AIDS. The difficulties that these workers have in supporting their claims are exacerbated by the industrial policies of the Thai government and the current economic crisis that seeks foreign capital investment at any cost.

In Cambodia, the garment industry has become a major export industry, with a large number of companies moving their operations there from other countries in the region, including Thailand. The production of cheap garments comes at a price for the workers of these factories. Like the workers described in the electronics industries of Thailand, they work long hours and earn low wages. Kasumi Nishigaya finds that many of the workers are unable to survive and support their families on the wages they earn in the factories, and so make decisions to supplement their incomes with sex work. This takes several forms, including brothel-based work, work within karaoke bars, or the more discretionary work of beer promoters. Through case studies of some of these women, Nishigaya documents the various gradients of power that affect women's health. Relations of power structure their experience as migrants, as workers in the factories or in the sex industry, and the cultural expectations that as daughters they will provide economic support for their rural families. Under these conditions, women appear to have limited means to protect themselves from HIV and other sexually-transmitted diseases. At the micro-level, gender subordination keeps women from negotiating the use of condoms with their 'guests' or 'sweethearts.' At the macro-level, it excludes unmarried garment factory workers from health programs to address HIV/AIDS. As Nishigaya notes, it is ironic that women sex workers, arguably some of the least powerful people in Cambodian society, are expected to be the promoters of condom use to protect the population from the spread of AIDS by their male clients and partners.

These themes of power and health also resonate through a set of papers dealing with reproductive health, which highlight the differences between women's own understandings and knowledge of their bodies, and the biomedical understandings reflected in health programs. As detailed in Maxine Whittaker's paper, health programs wishing to improve the diagnosis or treatment of reproductive tract infections (RTIs) in Vietnam, for example, need to understand the ways in which women define and treat their illnesses and the social meanings of RTIs. She presents us with insights into the significance of RTIs to women's experience of their health and bodies, something that has been too often overlooked in family planning and reproductive health programs. Worldwide, women suffer a substantial morbidity from such infections, but a culture of silence reigns over their pain, itching, malodorous discharge and discomfort during intercourse. All too often, health service providers fail to acknowledge these problems or are ill-equipped to deal appropriately with them. Women's treatment and care decisions are not just made on the basis of their symptoms, but are structured by considerations of their role as workers providing for their families, the ideological pressure to maintain family harmony, inadequate health services, the imperative to have small families, even a woman's social and religious positioning within the Vietnamese state. Health service providers' emphasis upon the role of dirt and germs in gynecological health lead them to blame women for their lack of hygiene. As a consequence, women suffering these problems may be reluctant to admit their symptoms to service providers. As Whittaker notes, poverty ensures that their health will remain problematic, due to the combined effects of unsanitary working conditions, poor nutrition, and poor living conditions.

The complexity of women's understandings of their reproductive health is also illustrated in the paper by Pimpawun Boonmongkon and her colleagues, reporting upon a large study of women's health problems in northeast Thailand. In parallel with M. Whittaker's paper, they explore women's definitions of their gynecological health. The womb and its flows are a focus for women's understandings of their health and well-being. Women fear cancer as the long-term consequence of problems they experience and the paper details the logic behind their fears. Boonmongkon and her colleagues' paper has important ramifications for the screening and prevention of cervical cancer. It describes the dangers in the introduction of a public health program that fails to take into account local understandings of gynecological health and its consequences. They argue that "global" health discourses and practices are transformed in "local" settings, often taking on new hybrid meanings. They also describe a positive example of research as a form of advocacy to inform and introduce more sensitive, holistic reproductive health services.

The final two papers also move beyond stereotypical concerns with family planning. Monique Skidmore writes of the multiple meanings of menstruation and menstrual regulation in Burma, placing her analysis of the experience of health firmly within the political context. As in the Thai paper by Boonmongkon et al., Skidmore argues that blood flow is a key symbol in women's definitions of well-being. The women with whom she works explain that body, mind and soul cannot be well unless the physical and spiritual context is harmonious. The current political regime with its enforced economic hardship jeopardizes this harmony. Weakness is a central idiom of distress in Burma, understood to cause potentially dangerous menstrual disorders which threaten women's sanity and even their life. The experience of psychiatric illness is thus understood and experienced through reproductive health. The continual worry and economic stress experienced by women struggling with poverty in relocated townships are manifested in the thriving market for "medicine for women's diseases."

Finally, my own work on abortion in Thailand highlights the effects of the government's current restrictive abortion laws. The situation in Thailand echoes that of many women throughout the world whose choices are limited by a lack of access to legal abortion services. Rural women in Thailand rarely have the resources necessary to access the safe clinical services operated illegally by doctors. Many resort to local methods, ranging from traditional massage abortions to the dangers of injection abortions by untrained practitioners. This paper also speaks briefly of the current advocacy work being undertaken in Thailand to amend the law. The experiences of Thai women undergoing illegal abortions reminds us of the ramifications of the recent stance taken by the Bush administration to reinstate the ban on family planning funds to international family planning groups that offer abortion or abortion counseling. His action highlights the global nature of the debate surrounding abortion and how political interventions by one country can have direct repercussions upon women's health in another.

As in any edited collection, the coverage of issues can only be partial. Within the region, there is still a paucity of research on issues such as domestic violence, sexual violence and abuse, chemical exposure of women in agricultural occupations, the gendered effects of drug and tobacco addiction in the region, and the introduction of new reproductive technologies. What the papers of this collection share is a focus on women's health within its social and cultural context. They witness the constraints placed upon women's agency by power relations and politics, the need for sensitivity to women's own desires and choices, the social and cultural meanings of their experiences, and how inequalities in health and access to services constitute a source of extreme gender discrimination. The collection provides an opportunity to reflect upon the indivisibility of women's health and their human rights. The women workers described in this volume suffer from the global political economy and gendered inequalities that place them at the bottom of the work hierarchy, with low wages and poor working conditions. The rights of women to physical integrity and personal security are threatened within the violent conditions of the Cambodian sex industry, or the state violence that is an oppressive threat to women in Burma. Reproductive rights to decide upon the number and spacing of their children are infringed by state policies that punish Vietnamese women (not men) for excess or mistimed fertility, or force women to have illegal abortions under Thailand's restrictive abortion laws. Ultimately, as women themselves remind us throughout the papers of this collection, poverty is intimately related to women's access to health. Women in poverty throughout the region have few choices to maintain their health. When illness does strike, it threatens their livelihoods and the security of their families.

The papers provide a glimpse of these issues from women's points of view in ways not possible through quantitative research methods. The women's voices throughout this collection invite us to learn more of their lives and become aware of the broader issues impinging upon their health.

Gendered Bodies:
Recruitment, Management
and Occupational Health
in Northern Thailand's Electronics Factories

Sally Theobald, PhD

SUMMARY. This paper explores workers' experiences and understandings of occupational health hazards in the electronics industries of northern Thailand. Women form the bulk of the lower-level workforce as operators responsible for assembling the parts that make up microchip components. Drawing data from 16 months of research in workers' dormitories, formal and informal interviews and questionnaire surveys, in this paper I explore how gender relations are central to the organization and experience of work in these industries. I identify "work process" health hazards resulting from the physical working environment, and "workplace" health hazards relating to the organizational and social pressures of the working environment. Musculoskeletal pain, eye strain, chemical exposure, stress, improper use of safety equipment and accidents all impact upon women workers' health. Additionally, risk behaviors such as

Sally Theobald is Lecturer in Social Science and International Health, School of Tropical Medicine, Pembroke Place, Liverpool, L3 5QA, UK (E-mail: sjt@liv.ac.uk).

The author would like to thank all the women workers in the Northern Regional Industrial Estate who shared their experiences, hopes and aspirations with her. The author would also like to thank her PhD supervisor, Professor Ruth Pearson, and Dr. Rhys Jenkins for their support during this research.

The author thanks the Leverhulme Trust and the University of East Anglia, UK for financial support.

[Haworth co-indexing entry note]: "Gendered Bodies: Recruitment, Management and Occupational Health in Northern Thailand's Electronics Factories." Theobald, Sally. Co-published simultaneously in *Women & Health* (The Haworth Medical Press, an imprint of The Haworth Press, Inc.) Vol. 35, No. 4, 2002, pp. 7-26; and: *Women's Health in Mainland Southeast Asia* (ed: Andrea Whittaker) The Haworth Medical Press, an imprint of The Haworth Press, Inc., 2002, pp. 7-26. Single or multiple copies of this article are available for a fee from The Haworth Document Delivery Service [1-800-HAWORTH, 9:00 a.m. - 5:00 p.m. (EST). E-mail address: getinfo@haworthpressinc.com].

amphetamine and alcohol use, and unprotected sex, are associated with
the social context of factory work. *[Article copies available for a fee from
The Haworth Document Delivery Service: 1-800-HAWORTH. E-mail address:
<getinfo@haworthpressinc.com> Website: <http://www.HaworthPress.com>
© 2002 by The Haworth Press, Inc. All rights reserved.]*

KEYWORDS. Gender, work, occupational health, electronics, Thailand

INTRODUCTION

Debates on gender, development and industrialization are largely
concerned with addressing the effects of participation on industrial assembly lines for women workers' lives and for patterns of gender identities and relationships. Are forms of gender subordination intensified,
recomposed or decomposed with the uptake of industrial work (Elson &
Pearson 1981:31)? With notable exceptions (Buakamsri 1996; Mills
1999), little research has been carried out investigating the effects of industrial work on Thai women's lives, even less on what such work
means for women workers' health. The academic and popular gaze on
women's work in Thailand is largely sexualized and exoticized (Pearson
and Theobald 1998). Any literature or Internet search on "women,"
"work" and "Thailand" will reveal tonnes of information on sex work
and sexually transmitted infections, but very little on industrial work
and occupational health. Yet, the female workforce has been fundamental to the growth of Thailand's industrial base, and in particular its export industries (Phongpaichit and Baker 1996; Bell 1997; Mills 1999).

This paper takes a qualitative worker-centered approach in investigating the extent and experience of occupational health hazards in the
Thai electronics industries. I explore how gender and hierarchy inter-
weave to shape the day and night working experiences of women workers in northern Thailand. I demonstrate how working practices and
processes in electronics industries constitute occupational health hazards and are profoundly gendered.

Since the mid-1980s, the Thai government has followed a strategy of
industrial decentralization and has established industrial estates outside
the congested Bangkok metropolis (Warr 1993; Thai Development
Newsletter 1996). The study on which this paper is based was conducted with workers from one such industrial estate–the Northern Regional Industrial Estate (NRIE) in Lamphun, constructed in 1985. The

NRIE is 30 kilometers south of Chiangmai, the regional capital of northern Thailand. Investors who located their industries in the NRIE have benefited from a set of investment incentives and privileges, infrastructural provision, an abundance of cheap female labor and the absence of trade unions[1] (interviews, NRIE staff office and factory representatives). There are currently 17 electronics factories operating in the NRIE (interview, NRIE office staff). The majority of these are Japanese-owned and produce electronic components for sale in a global market.

Most workers in the lower echelons in NRIE factories are women. Disaggregated employee data pertaining to sex and job classification was available for 1998 from nine[2] different factories. Only five women were employed at the well-paid management level out of a total of 109 positions. However, women predominate as low paid operators, who assemble and check the complex parts forming microchips. Out of a total of 8,517 operators, 7,482 were female and 1,035 were male. Why these gendered patterns exist demands an investigation of the specific demand and supply of female labor within the political economy of these global industries. The first part of this paper explores the role of gender within the demand for female labor. The second part explores the consequences for women's health in these settings.

METHODS

The methods used in this study included participatory observation while living in a workers' dormitory for 16 months, open conversations with workers, a series of informal interviews (both group and individual), key informant interviews and questionnaires (seventy completed questionnaires from women workers were analyzed). The sample was purposive. The majority of workers who participated in the research were female, age 18-26, and migrants from the north or northeast of Thailand. In addition, I was allowed to conduct interviews with factory representatives from eight of the seventeen electronics companies. All names of individuals in the paper are pseudonyms, although the factory names are real.

A FEMINIZED WORKFORCE

According to the representatives of NRIE factories, the ideal operator is a young, healthy, unmarried female with at least a primary education who is fast working. At one factory, this preference is taken to an extreme, with a company policy of employing only women as operators. This preference centers around essentialized notions of gender. Management representatives from 12 factories, and also 70 women workers, were asked why there is a preference for female operators. Their responses took two main forms. The first set of responses focused on women's physical make up: the fact that they are 'smaller' and 'neater' makes them suited to this assembly work, echoing trends described by Elson and Pearson (1981) of employers favoring women because of assumed psychological and physiological differences. One women worker from Murata explains, "This is very detailed work, women have small fingers, keen eyes and are more versatile–this is work for women." A Tokyo Coil management representative reinforces this: "Small and fiddly work requires small and dexterous workers–so we insist on young women."

In the NRIE, representations of women workers also make reference to the supposedly innate mental or social characteristics of women as more obedient, docile and motivated workers: "Women are more obedient than men–they respond and act on instructions" (management representative, Hana). An LTEC management representative explained:

> Women are more conscientious in sending remittances home to their family than men–this is part of our culture–it is how girls are brought up. This means that women are not only more reliable but that they will work harder in order to get more money to support their families.

The idea that women are more conscientious at work, in order to support their families, is derived from local patriarchal, socio-cultural and religious understandings of gender (see also Tonguthai 1987). Klausner (1997) explains that Thai women feel a particular financial filial obligation as, unlike their brothers, they cannot enter the monkhood and bring spiritual merit to their families. Testimonies from workers in the NRIE illustrate the importance of women's obligations to their families as a motivation to earn money. As one Murata worker explained, "Work in the NRIE means that I can bring money to my parents." A LTEC worker stated, "I came to the NRIE to look for work, in order to support my mother. My father has passed away and my brother is working abroad. He sends money sometimes. It is my duty to support my mother and I am happy to do it."

The expectation that daughters will contribute to their family budget facilitates the supply of female labor in the NRIE. In this way, local gender relations and cultural norms support the needs of global industry. All management representatives interviewed commented that the supply of female labor to fill the production lines has never been problematic, and that this has especially been the case during the recent economic crisis. This differs from South Asian contexts, for example, where women workers' visibility in public space transgresses socially specific cultural norms, and recruitment can be problematic (Kibria 1998).

As noted earlier, men are disproportionately more likely to be in supervisory and management positions. Operators work in groups of 10-15 and are controlled by a *huana line* (operator leader). *Huana line* in turn report to *supers* (supervisors), who are responsible to the lower echelons of the factory management. Where there are mixed operators, men are more likely to be promoted to *huana line* or *super* than women.[3] At Lamphun Shindegen and Namiki, factory representatives explained that approximately half the *huana line* and *supers* are male and half are female, despite the disproportionate number of women operators. On being questioned about this, factory representatives replied that men perform these sorts of jobs better–they can control the groups more efficiently; women will listen and respond to men. Efficiency in production is highly valued, and when a plant is stretched to full capacity, tension is likely to surface. Factory representatives feel that men can cope with this tension better than women. Gender representations of men as the controllers and leaders, and women as the passive order receivers, provide the logic behind management decisions related to efficiency.

CONCEPTUALIZING OCCUPATIONAL HEALTH

In examining occupational health hazards stemming from the electronics industry, I make the distinction between "work-process" and "workplace-related" occupational health hazards. This distinction is somewhat artificial, as the two types of hazards merge and overlap in workers' experiences. However, the distinction is useful in addressing the causes or triggers of occupational health hazards.

"Work-process" related hazards are the occupational health hazards usually referred to in the occupational health literature (Messing 1997). Such hazards stem from the physical, ergonomic, chemical and biological working environment–from repetitive and cumulative interaction with a particular work process. An example from the electronics indus-try is the job of some workers in quality control that involves bending over a high powered microscope to check that the final intermeshing of the intricate parts of a microchip is correct. This may result in eyestrain, bodily aches or repetitive strain injury (RSI). The work of other opera-tors involves interacting with chemicals such as solvents, and they may experience rashes or faintness.

"Workplace" occupational health hazards result from the social work-ing environment and relationships, and also from the regulations and expectations generated by the management. Hazards are also stress-re-lated, with triggers for stress embedded within the working environ-ment. As Craig (1991:20) argues:

> Stress can come from your job–bad work relations, violence and harassment, a grueling shift system, monotonous tasks, being pushed too hard or being expected to accomplish the impossible with faulty equipment, a poor communications set-up and con-flicting demands.

Within the electronics industry in Thailand, these occupational health hazards constitute a gendered phenomenon, as the labor force is re-cruited because of its perceived gender attributes. In addition, the rules and regulations that produce and sustain such hazards are negotiated along grids of power and hierarchy, in which gendered relationships play a crucial role.

WORK-PROCESS OCCUPATIONAL HEALTH HAZARDS

Operators in the NRIE are employed in producing microchips and other electronic components. Using machines and chemicals is an inte-gral part of the work process experienced by the majority of electronics operators in the NRIE. Although electronics industries globally are pro-moted as clean technology, as 'the pollution-free alternative to the gray smoke stacks of older industries' (Reardon 1994:1), the consequent health hazards of the processes involved have been wide reaching (Heng Leng 1994; Stuart 1994; Messing 1997; Ostlin 2000). The facto-ries that I visited did much to promote the image of pollution free cleanliness. Just to enter the administrative areas, I had to wear special shoes and a white coat in order to tread on the spotless floors, which were surrounded by walls covered with glossy pictures and phrases that boasted of the cleanliness, safety and modernity of the industry. The testimonies of workers from the same factories paint a very different picture.

Working with Machines:
'They Give Me an Aching Body and Sore Eyes'

Eighty-seven percent of the 70 currently employed workers who answered my questionnaire used a machine in their work. The main machine-riggered work process hazards are aching bodies and eye problems (strain, soreness, irritation and nearsightedness). From the questionnaire responses these two types of occupational health hazards were the most prevalent, with 80% of workers suffering from bodily aches and 60% experiencing eye problems (see Table 1).

Many workers also complained of stiffness and muscle soreness during and after work. Some experienced pain in their joints and wrists for protracted periods of time, which can be classed as musculoskeletal disorders. Workers often gave each other massages to try to alleviate some of the pain. A twenty-four year old Murata worker stated that:

> I have to weld the smallest component of the television and audio equipment. It is very detailed work and it hurts my arm from the machine used in the welding process and my eyes from the concentration. Sometimes I get migraines too from having to concentrate.

The boredom of repetitive tasks can also lead to injuries from the machines. Phaa, a 17 year old who had been working at Lamphun Shindegen for six months, explained:

> I work with a knife machine–it is very precise and used for cutting lenses. It is not really a dangerous machine, as it could not cut off my arm or my hand. But sometimes I get really bored just using it all the time that I drift away in my thoughts to keep amused and then sometimes I get cuts, like this one [shows cut on lower arm] when I was thinking of my mum back home in Nakhon Phayom.

Eye problems are a particular hazard for those working in quality control. Many explained that they have had to start wearing glasses for nearsightedness, whereas before they came to work in the NRIE their eyesight was good. Some joked about the linkage between length of

TABLE 1. Health Outcomes Related to Work Processes

Type of work process	Health outcomes	Percentage reporting problem (n = 70)
87% of workers used a machine	Bodily aches	80
	Eye problems	60
71% of workers used chemicals	Dizziness	53
	Numbness	26
	Rashes	26
	Fainting	23

time working with microscopes and the need for glasses. Some workers use lotions around their eyes to try to rest them and get rid of the redness.

Working with Chemicals: 'They Make Me Feel Faint'

Seventy-one percent of questionnaire respondents interacted with chemicals on a daily or nightly basis. For those workers, responses about their feelings while using and interacting with chemicals were entirely negative. Most of these responses centered around the smell of the chemical, or the pain/tingling experienced when it came into contact with the skin.

> I use a machine to check the specification of the product. My friends in the next room use the chemicals–I'm not sure what sort they are but I can smell them from where I stand. Some of my friends who work with the chemicals often get rashes on their arms which they say are painful and they have to try not to scratch them. (woman worker, LTEC)

Khwan, a 21 year old chip monitor worker, describes the process of her job and how it makes her feel:

> I must take the circuit plate on to the circuit board and then pour lead liquid on to the screen of the machine. The lead has a creamy grey color and stinks. I then expose dots of substance to the lead, if there is any problem in the process the plate must be considered defective and washed in a bucket of liquid. The liquid dissolves very rapidly, and if it reaches inside your nostrils you feel dizzy.

You then wash the product, it feels cold on the hand and is very painful on the skin and reaches deep into the bone. If your skin is exposed it turns white and peels off.

Jay worked at Tokyo Coil for over a year, three years ago. She was making small components that were then distributed around other sections of the factory. It was her first job, so there was no problem in getting it, as she was young and 'fresh faced' with no chemicals in her blood. Tokyo Coil pays for a doctor to come regularly to carry out a blood and general health check for all the workers:

> At first I had 8% of chemicals in my blood and then 24%. At 80% you die. The top *huana line* said I must be responsible for my health by myself otherwise I wouldn't be healthy enough to work anymore. I started to feel worse; I lost a lot of weight and was also fainting at work. My mother said I should quit. Since then I have to go to the doctor once a week and I must have injections and consume a lot of vitamins and sweet milk. I have to pay for the doctor visits and injections myself, it is very expensive.

The main chemically-triggered work process occupational health problems reported were weight loss, faintness, nausea, rashes, peeling skin, dizziness, numbness and headaches. Some workers have all of these symptoms, whereas others have only a few, depending on the chemicals used and the length of time worked. Information regarding the chemicals used and their effect on workers' bodies is problematic. As workers are not told the names of the chemicals they are working with, it is impossible to make a systematic correlation between chemical and effect. In the sample of 70 workers, 51% had experienced feelings of dizziness, 26% numbness, 26% had had rashes and 23% had fainted. The vignette from Jay illustrates the role of workers' own understandings about their health. Jay believes that with 80% of chemicals in your blood you must die. In a context where neutral and accessible information is rare, the role of rumors, misconceptions, fear and doubt is integral to the ways in which workers rationalize and internalize perceptions about their health.

Workers' testimonies show the complex, contradictory and ongoing relationship between themselves and their work. Women workers work physically *in* the NRIE–they travel in and out of the security areas of the industrial estate on a nightly or daily basis. The effects of this NRIE work can also be found physically and metaphorically *in* the bodies of women workers. Workers' bodies embody the chemicals in ways that mean their experience of work hazards goes with them beyond the factory gate.

WORKPLACE OCCUPATIONAL HEALTH HAZARDS

The production systems within these factories are geared towards maximizing efficiency and output. These also have implications for workers' health and well-being. In their analysis of management techniques in the Malaysian electronics industry, Heng Leng and Subramanian (1994:93) state that:

> The pressures placed upon the workers . . . are integral to how the work is organized. The electronics industry is very competitive, and the constant push for quality production at lower costs means that the management is always looking for ways in which work can be organized, and reorganized, so that productivity can be increased.

In the NRIE this organization and reorganization is placed within a *sawadtikan* framework. *Sawatdikan*, the variety of social welfare packages and rewards, combine to offer a range of carrot and stick type incentives and disincentives that are designed to facilitate the smooth running of the factory processes. *Sawatdikan* policies, negotiated and executed along gendered lines, combine to ensure maximum worker attendance and output at all times. *Sawatdikan* serve to complement the strict 24-hour operational regulations (relating to punctuality, toilet visits, appearance, etc.) that are in place in the factories. These processes combine to ensure maximum production and attendance, and place a heavy toll on workers (see Table 2).

Overtime and Night Shift

Workers in the factories typically work 12-hour shifts, punctuated by two or three breaks. Each week an average worker will work for six days, switching between night shift and day shift every week or fortnight. The long working hours with few breaks, and the alternating between day and night shifts, are detrimental to workers' health. Workers

TABLE 2. Health Outcomes Related to the Work Place Environment

Work place patterns	Common worker response	Health repercussions
Overtime and night shift	Long hours, alternating working patterns/hours	Exhaustion, interrupted sleep patterns and irregular periods, loss of appetite, guilt and stress related to interrupted familial and personal relationships
Diligence pay	A reluctance to take time off work when ill	Stress, exhaustion and poor recovery from sickness
Focus on maximum production (bonuses)	Intensive working patterns, missing lunch and other breaks, restricted toilet visits, internalization of blame, amphetamine intake, poor use of protective equipment	Exhaustion, aches and pains, swellings, stress, low self-esteem, interrupted sleep, amphetamine dependence, accidents inside and outside of the work place

complain of feeling exhausted, not being able to sleep properly, irregular menstrual cycles and appetite loss.

> My body finds it hard to adjust to a new working schedule. After two weeks when I switch to night shift I find I can't sleep in the day. It takes my body about five days to adjust and then before I know it it's back to day shift again and I can't sleep at night. (woman worker from LTEC)

> When I'm working on night shift I lose my appetite. I eat cakes and sweet things at night but I don't feel like a proper meal, although sometimes I manage one at 8 am. Then I feel myself getting really exhausted. (woman worker from Murata)

The shape and length of working days and working nights can also affect workers' personal relationships, resulting in feelings of guilt and stress. These workers described the disruption it causes to their social lives. As a KSS worker says, "When I'm on night shift I never get to see my boyfriend; I really miss him." A woman worker from LTEC explained, "It's difficult being a mother when you have to work these hours. Night shift is actually better as I get to see my kids after the nursery, but I'm normally tired then and don't feel like I give them my best which makes me feel guilty. My older sister looks after them for me."

Diligence Pay

An example of the *sawatdikan* policies that aggravate a stressful and unhealthy working environment is diligence pay. All factories have a system of diligence pay (*biakhayan*) that is designed to achieve maximum attendance. At Lamphun Shindegen, for example, operators receive a monthly bonus if they report at the factory every day on time, and this increases as punctuality continues. However, one late arrival means the loss of all accumulated bonuses.

Workers will go to great lengths to secure this wage increase. Operators report that such a system, although financially beneficial, places them under extreme stress. As I witnessed many times, this has repercussions for health, as workers will go to work even when seriously sick, to avoid jeopardizing their diligence pay. For example, when I asked a sick worker friend why she didn't take time off work, she replied:

> I went to work today and started to feel worse, I hope I get better tonight, as I have to go to work tomorrow. If I don't go I will lose my bonus. I have just got it up to 500 baht (US$12) and I can't lose it, as I want to go home next weekend.

Diligence pay pressures workers into coming to work regardless of their health. This not only exposes other workers to sickness, but also increases the likelihood of poor recovery, complications and workplace accidents.

Bonuses for Speed Gradation

The bonus system in the Thai-Japanese Electro-Ceramics factories groups workers into classes depending on their speed of output. Bonuses operate on a sliding scale, so that the fastest Class A workers get paid the most, and the slowest Class D workers the least. This system serves to increase output and maximize competition between workers, as only a certain number of workers can be awarded Class A status. Targets for production are also in place in many of the other factories, at both individual and group level. At Namike, groups are rewarded if they reach certain targets on a weekly level, and this produces group peer pressure to increase output and gain bonuses. As Cardoso-Khoo and Jin (1989:205) comment "This type of competition (at both individual and group levels) is a very effective psychological threat constantly hanging over the heads of workers."

The *sawatdikan* policy of grouping workers into classes by speed of output, and remunerating on a sliding scale, is also problematic in terms of workers' health. Electro-Ceramics workers comment that it is Class A operators who are more likely to get sick. One woman operator from Electro-Ceramics explains:

> I get so tired all the time trying to work fast so I can keep my 'A' status. I have to stand up to operate the knife cutting machine and I don't get a break for four hours in a row. It's really exhausting and my legs begin to hurt a lot and sometimes they swell up too but then they go down again after I have left the workplace and can relax and go to sleep.

There is continuous pressure on workers to perform quickly and to meet targets, which in turn respond to processes of global demand. This pressure is applied by the *huana line*, who in turn is pressured from above. At a group level there is intense peer pressure, encouraged by the group leader, for each member to work to their maximum capacity. Group dynamics in a scenario of maximum output can be very stressful, especially in a context of high worker turnover, where workers must keep readjusting to new members of their production line.

This pressured environment is reinforced by the hierarchical management structure. The power relations ensure that any delays in production are blamed on the lowest level staff, the operators. The operators explain that if there are problems in production, too many defects, or a machine is broken, the blame will eventually end up with them as no one else wants to take responsibility. This adds further to the stress of the work environment. As a woman operator from Lamphun Shindegen explained, "If something goes wrong and we are accused, what can we do? Often we take the blame even if it is not our fault. There is no way to answer to the accusations so we just stay silent." A Tokyo Try operator explained the ways in which she deals with technical faults,

> I am a coil worker, one coil takes 6.5 seconds and I am meant to make 5,500 pieces in one day. If there is a problem with the machine I use, for example the machine is broken or the power is switched off, I use my lunch time or breaks to try and cover up the problem, otherwise it will be seen as my fault and I will be blamed.

Amphetamine Intake

In the NRIE, some workers respond to the pressure for maximum production by taking stimulants to enhance their output. For example, Noy explains:

> I began taking tablets of *ya ma* (amphetamines) because they make me work quicker and get more bonuses. Now I do it every day, and sometimes take two or three tablets. If I don't take any tablets I feel unmotivated and can't work at all. It is common at my factory–sometimes we hide the tablets in our lipsticks. Other workers don't take tablets but drink energy drinks[4] many times a day and that enables them to work faster.

Some workers report difficulty in sleeping on days off, as the body becomes used to daily amphetamine intake. Olden (1997) states that amphetamines are capable of producing intense patterns of dependence, and can make users more vulnerable to a range of physical and psychological health conditions including muscle tremors and psychosis. Use of amphetamines, together with high levels of stress, long working hours and shift work, contributes to the gradual deterioration in a worker's health. It is likely that they can also contribute to workplace accidents, as a result of exhaustion.

Poor Use of Protective Equipment

In a working environment that rewards maximum output, both explicitly in terms of financial remuneration and implicitly in terms of approval, many workers decide to forgo using protective equipment as it hinders their speed. A Murata operator explains the dynamics in her group:

> We have gloves we can wear and also protective pieces to put over our mouths and noses–sometimes I wear them. I prefer to wear them as the smell is bad and after many hours I feel nauseous. But if we have a big order to meet and the pressure is on, they slow you down and there is a sort of group agreement not to wear the stuff so that we can all work quicker.

In the NRIE, most factory representatives interviewed insisted that all necessary protective equipment is provided and that it is compulsory to wear it. However, some workers stated that the equipment is not always available, or that after it becomes worn out it takes a while before it is replaced. Some factory representatives expressed their irritation over lack of use of protective equipment, for example:

> Workers just don't like to wear their protective equipment; they don't see why they should. It's just like when they ride their motorbikes, they don't wear their helmets. Now we are going to introduce a policy of penalizing workers who turn up to work without a motorbike helmet. (management representative, KSS)

It is illuminating that the penalties will be for non-wearing of motorbike helmets, rather than of protective equipment inside the factory, the use of which may slow down production–anathema to the maximum output factory ideology.

BEYOND THE WORKPLACE:
WIDER IMPLICATIONS

NRIE workers also face health risks posed by the situation outside the factory walls. The most obvious to an observer is the alarming frequency of motorbike accidents. Workers' networks with which I came into contact reported the motorbike accident deaths of three NRIE workers,[5] and many injuries.

A strong emphasis on punctuality, heavy traffic[6] at peak times, fatigue and in some cases the use of stimulants or alcohol all contribute to the risk of motorbike accidents. Thirty-five percent of women workers who responded to the questionnaire had been involved in a road accident since working in the NRIE. Most of these accidents occurred in the congested dormitory areas around the NRIE. Others took place as workers traveled long distances home to visit their families, having just completed a 12-hour night shift. The high incidence is also due to the geography of the area and the lack of physical infrastructure. The main areas of the NRIE lie on either side of the main motorway between Bangkok and Chiangmai, which carries heavy long distance traffic. Workers traveling from the NRIE into Lamphun city center must also cross a railway line. The smaller roads between the dormitories and markets are inadequately lit and badly maintained.

The less visible health risks are due to the lifestyle associated with factory work. Singhanetra-Renard (1995) discusses how workers in vulnerable situations, in which they are easily exploited in terms of wages, health and welfare, may engage in high-risk behavior. In the context of the Thai construction industry, she states that workers' health problems are aggravated by indiscriminate sexual behavior, and the regular use of analgesics, alcohol and commercially available stimulants.

Similarly, some NRIE workers have lifestyles outside factory working hours that are problematic for their health. Risk behaviors include high levels of alcohol intake, drug use, inadequate sleep and unprotected sex. For some workers, participating in such activities is an expression of freedom and financial independence–doing things they wouldn't be able to do easily back in their home villages. For other workers, inebriation offers a form of escapism–a way to forget the frustration and stresses of the workplace, as one woman operator explains: "After six long days of work, I feel exhausted, stressed and irritable. Getting wasted [drinking lots of whisky] is a way to forget it all and to relax."

On Sundays in my dormitory, some workers would drink excessive alcohol to the point of vomiting. Drinking and drug use is gendered in that more men than women indulge in such activities. However, drinking by women is seen as especially problematic by many of the local Lamphun residents. Along with casual sex, these behaviors triggered much consternation on the part of dormitory owners, who bemoaned the corruption of morality brought about by industrialization. Some dormitory owners claim that women workers desperate for money practice prostitution in their dormitories (Buakamsri 1996).

It is likely that stories of women's behavior that transcend gendered notions of acceptability and appropriateness in the Thai context are exaggerated by factory owners and government representatives alike. The large majority of women workers did not appear to engage in high risk behaviors. However my own research, that of Buakamsri (1996) and testimonies from women workers at the annual planning meeting for the Lamphun Women's Health Center in January 2001, suggest that workers experience unplanned pregnancies resulting from unprotected casual sex. Women in this situation resort to illegal abortions, sometimes with untrained practitioners (see Whittaker, A. this volume).

Unprotected sex also puts women at risk of STDs and HIV/AIDS. Anecdotal evidence from LTEC officials suggest that rates of HIV seropositivity are increasing annually amongst their workers, reflecting a general trend amongst young Thai women. In 1997 there were 2,930 AIDS cases amongst women of the 20-29 age group; in 1998, this number had risen to 3,103 (UNAIDS/WHO 2000). High-risk lifestyles engaged in due to their novelty value, or as a means to escape the tedious and stressful realities of the workplace, do undoubtedly have health repercussions. However, it is also arguable that these repercussions, namely HIV/AIDS, are focused on and exaggerated as a way of diverting attention and analysis away from occupational health hazards, which stem more directly from work processes. For example, one government official blamed sickness in women NRIE workers upon their sexual behaviors: "You have to understand these are young rural women, living in the city, away from their parents for the first time. Sometimes they are sexually irresponsible and AIDS is the result." Similarly, a factory representative commented that sickness is likely to be due to women operators' inability to look after themselves: "These young women are inexperienced and naive, they go to the discos till late at night, they don't eat enough or get enough sleep. They have casual sex. Sexually transmitted diseases and exhaustion are the result."

HIV and AIDS constitute a perfect scapegoat for occupational health hazards. Indeed, HIV/AIDS and solvent/chemical poisoning can manifest themselves in similar ways, with body wasting, ulcers and rashes. In the early 1990s, sickness and mortality rates amongst NRIE workers received considerable attention. For example, the *Bangkok Post* (Anon. 1994a, b, c), declared that between 11 and 23 people died from work-related causes in the NRIE up to 1994. Controversy surrounding sickness and deaths in the NRIE has reverberated around Thailand through various media, including newspapers, radio, word of mouth and popular music. In response to this development, IEAT called a conference in 1993 in an attempt to clear the NRIE's reputation with respect to safety standards The IEAT Governor, Dr. Thinapong, together with the Lamphun Health Authority, blamed the deaths on AIDS.[7] Occupational health specialist Dr. Orapan Methadigokul claims that there is a severe lack of evidence for attributing the deaths to HIV/AIDS, and that such a testimony constitutes "a most shameful reflection on the medical society" (Anon. 1994b).

CONCLUSIONS

A range of occupational health hazards face workers in the rapidly expanding electronics industry. These hazards are gendered, both because of selective recruitment practices of the factories and the ways in which work is organized. Using the stories of women workers in the

NRIE, this paper explores the work process and workplace based components of occupational health hazards, detailing the multiplicity of their causality. For many workers, the interface between workplace and work process occupational health hazards is inextricably linked in numerous and complex ways. This overlap keeps us focused on the need for a holistic analysis, and on the importance of incorporating psychosocial and workplace relationships into studies on occupational health.

Occupational health hazards constitute serious health problems for women workers across the globe. These hazards are often neglected and discounted by factory owners, government officials and health professionals. Comprehensive and gender sensitive research needs to be carried out in a facilitatory and participatory manner, so that workers will have access to information about the implications of their work for their health and that of their future children. However, even with good information, many women in Lamphun will continue to risk their health to serve the global demand for electronic products, due to individual, familial and filial expectations. This situation is exacerbated by the lack of alternative employment options, with the Thai economic crisis producing redundancies in other industries.

NOTES

1. In the sparse literature on Thai trade unions, there is no mention of unions operating outside Bangkok and the eastern seaboard. See Hewison and Brown (1994) for commentary on the reasons behind the low percentage of union participation in the Thai workforce, and Theobald (1999) for a discussion of alternative organizational forms operating in the NRIE.

2. These factories are as follows: Tokyo Try, Thai Asahi, Tokyo Coil, Schaffner, Lamphun Shindegen, Hana, LTEC, Tohuko Oki and Namiki.

3. An exception is Tokyo Coil which has a company policy specifying that all operators and all *huana line* are women.

4. These are drinks that contain a high proportion of caffeine.

5. Official statistics on traffic accident deaths were not available, although one official commented that they were very high.

6. The large majority of workers own a motorbike on which they travel to and from work. Most factories' shifts are from 8 a.m. to 8 p.m., and from 8 p.m. to 8 a.m., so at these turn-over times traffic is very dense.

7. Carabou, one of Thailand's most popular folk bands, wrote a song entitled 'Lamphun,' which details the environmental and health repercussions of Japanese electronics factories in the NRIE.

REFERENCES

Anon. (1994a). Suspicious deaths and illnesses of workers to be investigated, *Bangkok Post,* February, 25, p. 8.

Anon. (1994b). Lamphun factories face probe, *Bangkok Post,* March 1, p. 7.

Anon. (1994c). More deaths occur at NRIE, *Bangkok Post,* 27 May, p. 5.

Bell, P. (1997). Thailand's economic miracle: Built on the backs of women. In V. Somswasdi and S. Theobald (eds.). *Women, gender relations and development in Thai society.* Chiang Mai: Women's Studies Center, Faculty of Social Sciences, Chiang Mai University.

Buakamsri, T. (1996). Spatial mobility and health risks among factory workers in the Northern Regional Industrial Estate. Chiang Mai: MA Dissertation, Department of Geography, Chiang Mai University.

Cardoso-Khoo, J. and Khoo, K.J. (1989). Work and consciousness: Women workers in the electronics industry in Malaysia. In K.Young (ed.) *Serving two masters: Third world women in development.* Ahmedabad: Allied Publishers Ltd.

Craig, M. (1991). *Office workers' survival handbook–fighting health hazards in the office.* London: The Women's Press.

Elson, D. and R. Pearson (1981). Nimble fingers make cheap workers, *Feminist Review,* 7: 87-107.

Heng Leng, C. (1994). Introduction. In C. Heng Leng (ed.) *Behind the chip: Proceedings of the conference on safety and health in electronics,* Petaling Jaya, Malaysia, December 1992, Petaling Jaya: Women's Development Collective & Persatuan Sahabat Wanita.

Heng Leng, C. and M. Subramanian. (1994). Speaking out: women workers talk about safety and health in the workplace. In C. Heng Leng (ed.) *Behind the chip: Proceedings of the conference on safety and health in electronics,* Petaling Jaya, Malaysia, December 1992. Petaling Jaya: Women's Development Collective & Persatuan Sahabat Wanita.

Hewison K. and A. Brown. (1994). Labour and unions in an industrialising Thailand, *Journal of Contemporary Asia,* 24(4): 483-514.

Kibria, N. (1998). *Becoming a garments worker: The mobilization of women into the garments factories of Bangladesh.* Geneva: United Nations Research Institute for Social Development, UNRISD.

Klausner, W. (1997). *Thai culture in transition.* Bangkok, Amarin Printing and Publishing Public Company Limited.

Mills, M.B. (1999). *Thai Women in the global labour force.* New Jersey: Rutgers University Press.

Messing, K. (1997). Women's occupational health: A critical review and discussion of current issues, *Women and Health,* 25(4): 37-68.

Olden, K. (1997). Substance abuse and employee assistance programs. In J. Ladou (ed.) *Occupational and environmental medicine.* Hemel, Hempstead: Appleton & Large.

Ostlin, P. (2000). Gender inequalities in occupational health. Working Paper Series, 10(9), September, 2000. Boston: Harvard Centre for Population and Development Studies, Harvard School of Public Health, Harvard University.

Pearson, R. and S. Theobald. (1998). From export processing to erogenous zones: International discourses on women's work in Thailand, *Millennium: Journal of International Studies*, 27(4): 983-993.

Phongpaichit, P. and C. Baker. (1996). *Thailand's boom*. Chiang Mai: Silkworm Books.

Reardon, G. (1994). Women and the global economy, industrial hazards and the international division of labour. Working paper, Manchester: Women Working Worldwide.

Singhanetra-Renard, A. (1995). Migration and the quality of life: The case of construction workers in Chiangmai job sites. Unpublished paper, Chiang Mai: Geography Department, Chiangmai University.

Stuart, P. (1994). Laws are not enough: The role of health and safety legislation in the UK (with special reference to the electronics industry). In C. Heng Leng (ed.) *Behind the chip: Proceedings of the conference on safety and health in electronics*, Petaling Jaya, Malaysia, December 1992. Petaling Jaya: Women's Development Collective & Persatuan Sahabat Wanita.

Thailand Development Newsletter. (1996). Industrial Estates expansion pushed all over Thailand, *Thailand Development Newsletter*, 31: 72

Theobald, S. (1999). Embodied Contradictions: Organising around Gender and Health Interests in the Electronics Industries of Northern Thailand. Unpublished PhD Thesis, Norwich: Department of Development Studies, University of East Anglia.

Tonguthai, P. (1987). Women and work in the Thailand and the Philippines. In ESCAP (ed.) *Women and economic participation in Asia and the Pacific*. Bangkok: United Nations Economic and Social Commission for Asia and the Pacific.

UNAIDS/WHO. (2000). Epidemiological Fact Sheet. HIV/AIDS and STIs in Thailand. Geneva: UNAIDS/WHO.

Warr, P. (1993). The Thai economy. In P. Warr (ed.) *The Thai economy in transition*. Cambridge: Cambridge University Press.

Female Garment Factory Workers in Cambodia: Migration, Sex Work and HIV/AIDS

Kasumi Nishigaya, MA

SUMMARY. Female garment factory workers in Cambodia are more exposed to HIV/AIDS than previously thought. Although HIV/AIDS epidemics are fast spreading in Cambodia, relatively little is known about

Kasumi Nishigaya is a PhD candidate, National Centre for Epidemiology and Population Health, Australian National University, ACT 0200, Australia (E-mail: Kasumi. Nishigaya@anu.edu.au). The author previously worked as Gender and Development Advisor of JICA in Tokyo and Cambodia, and Associate Expert funded by the Government of Japan in UNHCR Bangladesh.

The author would like to acknowledge her supervisors, Professor John Caldwell, Gabriele Bammer and Dorothy Broom of the National Center of Epidemiology and Population Health (NCEPH), the Australian National University. The author also wishes to express special appreciation to Barbara Fitzgerald (Country Representative), Lim Sok San, Kong Sowath, Pry Phally Phuong and Ly Kim Song (national staff) of APHEDA, who hosted her during field research in Cambodia. The author acknowledges that this research would not have been possible without the coordination support provided by Chuon Mon Thol and ten interviewers: Sok Thach, Sloth Sokhontheavy, Yim Sothun, Sok Simontha, Sen Sokuntheary, Suong Sotheavy, Kheng Ravy, Va Muonglida, Ul Bophuong and Khuon Miyouvoan. The author also acknowledges formal authorization from the National Centre for HIV/AIDS, Dermatology and STDs to use the database of sentinel surveillance and behavior surveillance. The author wishes to express special thanks to Dr. Hor Bun Leng for his facilitation. The author also expresses appreciation to the 1,000 garment factory workers whose active involvement in the research processes made this research possible.

The NCEPH fully funded the author's six months of field research.

[Haworth co-indexing entry note]: "Female Garment Factory Workers in Cambodia: Migration, Sex Work and HIV/AIDS." Nishigaya, Kasumi. Co-published simultaneously in *Women & Health* (The Haworth Medical Press, an imprint of The Haworth Press, Inc.) Vol. 35, No. 4, 2002, pp. 27-42; and: *Women's Health in Mainland Southeast Asia* (ed: Andrea Whittaker) The Haworth Medical Press, an imprint of The Haworth Press, Inc., 2002, pp. 27-42. Single or multiple copies of this article are available for a fee from The Haworth Document Delivery Service [1-800-HAWORTH, 9:00 a.m. - 5:00 p.m. (EST). E-mail address: getinfo@haworthpressinc.com].

27

the sexual health of women other than those perceived as commercial sex workers or married women of reproductive age. In-depth interviews with 20 unmarried female garment factory workers, who reported to have engaged in multi-partnered sex through direct or discretionary commercial sex occupations, demonstrate that they are exposed to HIV-risk created along the gradients of power. Low socioeconomic status (low education, meager factory wage and high dependency rate at their rural households) and obligations as daughters to provide for the family mainly determine their entry into sex work. At the location of sex work, they are subjected to physical violence, alcohol and drug use, both self-taken and forced, and receive meager wages. In a society where women are expected to be virtuous and obedient to parents and husbands, these workers are motivated to identify male sex partners in paid sex as "sweethearts" rather than "guests." These factors contribute to low consistency of condom use. This paper demonstrates the complex interrelationships between power, cultural definitions of intimacy and economic dependency, which structure sexual relationships and the risk of HIV/AIDS. *[Article copies available for a fee from The Haworth Document Delivery Service: 1-800-HAWORTH. E-mail address: <getinfo@haworthpressinc. com> Website: <http://www.HaworthPress.com> © 2002 by The Haworth Press, Inc. All rights reserved.]*

KEYWORDS. HIV/AIDS, migration, garment industry, Cambodia, youth

INTRODUCTION

HIV is spreading along "the gradients of power" constantly created and recreated by broad political, economic and social forces (Farmer 1999). Migrants in the Indochina region, like their contemporaries in other parts of the world, are recognized to be placed at much greater risk of HIV/AIDS than non-migrants. Their physical and social distance from familial and community support and control often results in changes in their identities and behavior patterns in their new contexts (Ford and Kittisuksathit 1996a), including drug and alcohol use and unprotected sex. Gender and youth add to the vulnerability of female migrants, who are expected to earn an income for their family with limited social skills and education (Farmer 1999; Ford and Kittisuksathit 1996b; Schoepf 1992). In the mainstream AIDS policy discourses, women are usually targeted either as commercial sex workers or as married women of reproductive age. These overlook the circumstances of the majority of the young female population (Caravano 1994). As young unmarried women form a large segment of the workforce in export-oriented industries and other service industries in the region, their omission raises serious concerns in terms of the social and economic impacts of HIV/AIDS.

Cambodia was once a war-torn country subject to proxy wars during the Cold War, and isolated from the rest of the world during the ruthless rule of the Khmer Rouge and during the Vietnamese occupation. But it has become reintegrated into the international community since 1991 following the Paris Peace Accord. Since the United Nations supervised election in 1994, Cambodia has followed a democratic model of governance and a market-driven economy under the advice of the International Monetary Fund. The garment manufacturing industry is the largest foreign currency earner at present. It has expanded rapidly due to the attraction of a cheap labor force and Most Favored Nation status given to Cambodia by the World Trade Organization, and the generalized system of preference or export quotas given bilaterally by OECD nations, most importantly by the United States of America (Hall 1999). As in other Asian countries, the garment industry is dominated by overseas Chinese capital due to a generous foreign investment policy and relatively relaxed government administration. Approximately 85% of its 189 factories are located in Cambodia's capital city, Phnom Penh. These factories prefer to employ young female rural migrants for their nimble hands, docility, and cheap labor cost, and attract considerable rural-urban migration (Hall 1999, cf. Theobald, this volume).

Cambodian women have always been economically active and are considered to enjoy more autonomy than their contemporaries in other Asian regions (Ledgerwood 1994). There has also always been a strong parental expectation that daughters should provide for the family. In the modern economy this takes a pragmatic form in daughters' increased mobility, evidenced in their urban migration into the garment manufacturing industry on a large scale (approximately 135,000 persons) (Garment Manufacturers Association Cambodia 1999; Ministry of Commerce 1999).

Expected codes of sexual conduct differ according to gender. Whereas men are culturally sanctioned to have more than one partner before and outside marriage, women are expected to be virgins until their marriage, and faithful to their husbands. Traditional Khmer ideals of virtuous women (*srey grab lekkana*) within Khmer literature and in the *chhabap srey* (literally 'women's code') are reinforced through education from mother to daughter (Ledgerwood 1994). Although prostitution is constitutionally illegal, sexual double standards for men and women mean that commercial sex is tolerated (Gorbach 1998). Since the arrival of the United Nations missions in the early 1990s, Cambodia has experienced a rapid spread of HIV/AIDS, with approximately 3% of the country's population estimated to be infected. The major mode of transmission is heterosexual with the highest rate of prevalence found in brothel-based commercial sex workers (approximately 50% in the 1999 HIV sentinel surveillance), followed by their major clients, police and military personnel (approximately 7-8%) (Samrith and Vonthanak 1998). A behavior surveillance survey also reported frequent risky sexual behavior by brothel-based commercial sex workers, police, the military, and female beer sales promoters (Gorbach 1998). As in other countries, there is a tendency in the mainstream AIDS policy and program discourses in Cambodia to dichotomize the female population into sex workers and married women (Sopheab et al. 1999). Young never-married female youths are simply overlooked as they are assumed to be sexually docile and there is strong cultural resistance to questioning their sexual activities.

Nevertheless, there are numerous reports about sexual activities by young never-married females prior to marriage and outside the commercial sex industry (CARE 1998). In this paper, I draw upon narratives from 20 case studies of female garment factory workers who reported themselves in a survey as having engaged in sex with multiple partners (hereafter referred to as multi-partnered sex) in the previous week. I explore reasons why they engage in multi-partnered sex, illustrate their working conditions, and consider their position in the age of the AIDS epidemic.

METHODS

Findings in this paper are derived from my field study, conducted January-June 2000, which aimed to explore the sexual lifestyles and influencing factors of female garment factory workers in Phnom Penh. Three research methods were used in my field study: (1) focus group discussions to explore determinants of factory employment and evolving sexual cultures among garment factory workers (n = 75, 5 persons per group, 15 groups); (2) a quantitative survey (face-to-face and structured) on socio-demographic background, working conditions, leisure activities, sexual experience and health issues (n = 852, never-married and age less than 24 or equal to 24 years old); and (3) in-depth interviews on multi-partnered sex (n = 20, selected with consent from the respondents in the structured interviews). In the quantitative survey, 466 persons (54.6%) reported to have experienced vaginal sexual intercourse during the previous twelve months. Among them, 42 persons (4.9% of the sample population, 9.0% of sexually experienced respondents) reported to have engaged in multi-partnered sex during the previous week through various sex occupations. In the in-depth interviews (semi-structured), on which this paper draws, I explored reasons for this.

As I was primarily interested in how women workers articulate their own personal experience, an issue in the research design was with who, how and where I conduct my research. The existing literature in sexual behavior research in Cambodia tends to emphasize the matching of the sex of interviewers and respondents (Sopheab et al. 1999). I also felt it necessary to match the socio-economic class status of the interviewers and respondents, given that the majority of Cambodia's female workers are located at the bottom of the global garment production chain as machine operators (Nishigaya 1999) and that Khmer society is hierarchical in nature and characterized by vertical patron-client relationships (Chandler 1993). Accordingly, I worked with ten former or current women workers as research assistants. An Australian NGO, Australian People for Health, Education and Development Abroad (APHEDA), hosted my stay and provided technical help in training research assistants, translation and interpretation. I included only machine operators in the sample and recruited women workers outside the factory gate where they emerged to the street after work. All interviews were conducted at a location external to their workplace during their free time.

The research was limited to Phnom Penh, where most garment factories are located. Women constitute the majority of the workforce in this industry (approximately 90%) (Garment Manufacturers Association Cambodia 1999; Department of Labor Inspection 1999; Ministry of Commerce 1999). Most are clustered in the job category of machine operators (sewing, knitting, overlocking and ironing), located at the bottom of the global garment production hierarchy.

Demographic and Socioeconomic Profile of the Respondents

Most women who reported working in the sex industry come from rural households with less than one hectare of rice land, insufficient to support a family. They usually have little or no education (often primary school education was not completed). They are supporting many younger siblings who need education. They often come from single parent families (usually female-headed households). For example, Kimtouch, a never-married worker, is 24 years old. She came from a province of the central plain region where people engage in subsistence-level rice-farming. With three other younger sisters and brothers, she was brought up solely by her mother; her father was killed during the Khmer Rouge regime. As a widow who lacked male labor power for rice-farming, Kimtouch's mother took up extra work to earn the family's food, planting and cropping rice for other families in the village and engaging in petty trading. These represent two major income earning activities by rural women in Cambodia. The family rice field was sold in the early 1990s when the family needed cash for her mother's hospitalization. Due to the economic pressure since early childhood, Kimtouch could study only two years in elementary school. As her mother became older, Kimtouch needed to provide for her younger sisters and brothers.

Kimtouch's story of poverty and responsibility for her family was repeated across my sample. Many of the women come from the central plain region. This area has the highest population density in Cambodia and is prone to natural calamities such as drought and excessive floods. The economic changes caused by the new market economy have brought greater need for cash income to pay for services and education. Meanwhile, the market price of rice, the only income source of the majority of Cambodians, has remained low. There is increased pressure upon daughters to earn cash income for the family.

The pressure for cash can become acute when families experience a crisis, as in the case of Kimtouch's mother's illness. Lida, a 23 years old worker, also comes from a province of the central plain region. Her family lives in a small house made of thatch, the building material of the very poor, and owns less than one hectare of rice field due to repeated division of the land for inheritance. Since the early 1990s, Lida's father has worked as a cyclo-driver in Phnom Penh to gain cash income for the family. He now lives with his second wife in Phnom Penh, and hardly comes back to the family. Lida was brought up only by her mother, and could finish only three years of schooling. Her mother no longer works, as a consequence of a stroke. Among eight brothers and sisters, Lida is the only one who earns cash income at present from factory employment. Four younger brothers and sisters need support for their education. The elder brothers cannot support them as their earnings from rice-farming are nominal.

Women's Involvement in Sex Work

Women workers cite their low monthly wages from the factories as the main reason for their entry into sex work, although some report their abandonment by sweethearts (*sangsar*) who provided them with cash regularly. The heavy dependency ratio in rural households, expectations for daughters to provide support and the high living costs in Phnom Penh influence their entry into sex work. There are a variety of forms of sex occupations in Cambodia. Discretionary forms of sex work, as opposed to brothel-based sex work, have become widespread as they avoid public attention and include karaoke singers who accompany guests, and beer promoters who directly outreach customers at the restaurants to sell beer. Other forms of discretionary sex work reported by women workers involve working as night club dancers and bar attendants.

Sambo is 18 years old. She started to work in a guesthouse after her day-shifts in the factory, which is located in the red-light area of Phnom Penh. Her monthly salary from the factory is only US$30, which is less than the legal minimum wage of US$40 stipulated under the Cambodia Labour Code of 1996. Her monthly wage is just enough to keep herself in Phnom Penh, where a shared room costs US$5 per person a month, while her food and water costs an additional US$20 per month. Money also needs to be found for her other costs like moto-taxi, electricity and clothes.

> Usually, I have no money at the end of each month. I needed to work as a [brothel-based] sex worker to feed my mother and young brothers and sisters in the village. As they farm [rice], they have no cash. . . I knew no other skills but the "sex business" to help the family.

Wii, who is 20 years old, started to sing at a karaoke parlor, ever since her third sweetheart left her for another woman. He used to provide some financial support to her every week in the form of five dollars' cash and food. She now takes guests for money every night. She earns US$35 from her garment factory work as she is still regarded to be on-the-job training. She stated that she needed to do "guest service,"

> Because in the middle of the month, I had no cash left. I had to force myself to have sex with guests who come to a restaurant I work in. I hate the job. I decided to work like this because my fam-

ily is so poor. My younger brothers and sisters [three altogether] are still studying. My elder brother is already married, but he only looks after his family. My parents are rice farmers, and very poor. They live in a tiny thatched house in the village. So, I decided to sing at night and sleep with guests for money after work. That way, I can send some money to my mother.

WORK CONDITIONS IN THE SEX INDUSTRY

Women report varying degrees of autonomy in their ability to decide when, where and with whom they have sex. Generally speaking, women working in brothels, guesthouses and karaoke parlors have less autonomy than those working as beer promoters. This is reflected in their descriptions of the men they have sex with during their sex work. Women in the former category call them "guests," the latter women call them "sweethearts," a term that denotes more intimacy than "guests." As the following narratives reveal, many women working in these establishments are subject to violence and coercion, forced drug and alcohol use, and frequently are cheated of their earnings. Their lack of power in their working conditions and sexual relations places them at high risk of unprotected sex and hence HIV/AIDS infection.

Violence Against Workers

Physical violence against workers within sex establishments was common. Perpetrators were reported to be karaoke shop-owners, brothel-owners, restaurant-owners, and guests. They exercise violence against workers for a variety of reasons. Kimtouch, a karaoke singer, explains: "When I am paid little by guests, employers [karaoke owners] become very angry. They shout and spit into my face. Because I receive little, I can pay little to them. Then they lose their temper, and start shouting and slapping me."

Apart from disputes over money, women reported being coerced to have sex with guests. Pheap said, "The owner of the karaoke bar forces me to take guests. When I said I can't, they forced me by kicking my shins hard." Navi, another karaoke singer said, "The owner of the karaoke bar forces me to have sex with guests. If I say I do not want to, he slaps me in my face. He demands me to take guests every night." Generally speaking, workers feel as though there is no other option but to comply with the demands of their boss.

In contrast to the experience of women in brothels and karaoke parlors, beer sales promoters report neither physical violence nor coercion
by clients and/or guests and describe relative autonomy in the decision-making to take guests. Serey, a beer sales promoter, sleeps regularly with three "sweethearts" whom she met during her work at a
restaurant.

> After eight o'clock in the evening, I go to work as a "beer girl"
> (*lanse sra beer*). Before our departure from the company [by bus]
> every day, managers remind us to sell ten or twenty boxes of beers
> every month in order for us to get bonuses. If I cannot sell them, I
> simply do not get these bonuses . . . but no one forces me to have
> sex with guests [in the restaurants]. I only go out [with them] if I
> like them and if they like me. Normally, my sweethearts give me
> five dollars per meeting.

Drug Use

Some workers reported that they were forced to take drugs by guests
or proprietors before sex. In general, they know little about the purposes
and effects of these drugs. Navin said that some of her karaoke parlor
guests mixed 'power drugs' with beer that they made her drink before
sex. Ountouch, another karaoke singer, stated,

> It is the owner of the karaoke bar who gives us drugs. She tells us
> to take drinks, which have drugs in it. But I do not know what they
> are. I do not want them at all because I am too afraid. But they sim-
> ply put drugs [tablets] in beer, and tell us to take it . . . [after that] I
> feel restless. I want to cuddle men all the time. I feel like taking
> guests.

Serey, a beer sales promoter, reported drug use by guests, but denied
using them herself. "Quite often guests take them [with beer] before
sex, and they also ask me to take them. One guest said if I took this drug,
I would feel like really loving him. But I have never taken them." A total
of nine workers in the quantitative survey reported drug use either consumed by themselves or through coercion, and among them six workers
reported multi-partnered sex. Generally speaking, they were reluctant
to describe details of the way they were given drugs.

Sex Fees

Sex fees charged to the guests and the fraction of commission taken away by proprietors vary from one location to another and from one occupation to another. Despite their "guest services," sometimes workers are not paid, or paid a marginal "fixed monthly wage" no matter how many guests they take for sex. Toun, an iron operator of a factory in the red-light area, works at a brothel at night. She reported, "No matter how many men I sleep with, I am paid only twenty dollars a month. Last Sunday, I even had ten guests. Absolutely disgusting." The government reported that the average sex fee that brothel-based sex workers receive is approximately 2,000 riel (approximately US$0.53), which is about half of the total charge to the guests (Gorbach 1998).

In some cases, men do not pay for the sexual services and workers have little power to force them to pay. As Ountouch, a karaoke singer, described, "Sometimes guests did not pay me after sex. They simply walked out." Thida, another karaoke singer, reported similar experiences: "Some guests take me to the guesthouse [to sleep], but did not pay the sex fee to me. They only paid the guesthouse charge and simply told me to get lost . . . or worse, my employer (karaoke and guesthouse owner) cuts down my salary, too. He does not believe that the guest cheated me."

Accounts by beer sales promoters suggest that they may be more likely to find wealthier partners who support them on a regular basis. When she was asked how much she was paid after she received guests for sex, Rin, a beer sales promoter, replied, "I did not get money for sex as they are my sweethearts. We are not like [brothel-based] sex workers." Nevertheless, she said that her current sweetheart, a driver in the same beer company, gives her US$50 a month. When they go out, most expenses are also covered by him.

RELATIONSHIPS WITH SWEETHEARTS

Apart from the "guests" with whom women have sex for money, many also have sex with their "sweethearts" who support them regularly. The term "sweetheart" denotes a more intimate regular relationship, but it usually also involves financial support. Ountouch has been pursued by a married man for some time. He has taken her out to local resorts where they eat special food and relax. One day, they went out to a resort along the river and rented a private room. Suddenly, she alleged, he "took over my body (*chap bangkom*)." After the event, he gave her US$15. Ever since then, she has been seeing him regularly at her room, which has been set up and paid by him. He gives her 10,000 riel (approximately US$3) every week. Toun, a brothel-based sex worker, had a sweetheart five months ago who worked in the same factory. They went out on Khmer New Years Days to a resort, where they had sex. Before their departure from the resort, he gave her US$5. While none of the women described sweetheart relationships as explicitly economic, they expect sweethearts to be financially supportive.

Kim Touch identifies her current partner (her third, another garment factory worker) as her sweetheart and explained why: "Because he loves me and . . . we get on well. I trust him and he gives me money also, he takes me out and pays for food, and he loves me a lot. So, I thought I can go out with him."

Navin met her current sweetheart at a ceremony in her native village. When she was asked why she considered him a sweetheart, she replied, "Because he loves me, and he says he loves me for ever and will take me as his future wife. He supports me [by money], and so I love him." Serey's sweetheart is a policeman, whom she met when she was selling fruit juice on the street. In comparing differences between her sweetheart and her casual sex friends (mostly university friends) "who come and go," she described, "When I go out with my sweetheart [to sleep with him], he gives me money. But others [university students] did not. They intended to cheat me. They did not give me a penny." Sambo, a brothel based sex worker, identifies her three regular guests as sweethearts: "They [carpenters] come [to the brothel] regularly to see me for paid sex. They like me as I am good at talking. I get on well with them, and I do not take money when they are not paid well."

CONDOM USE

The male partners of the women come from all walks of life. However, most are factory workers and moto-taxi drivers, are usually older than the women, and are sexually experienced. Recent government surveys report that 57.3% of the military, 51% of the police and 55.5% of the moto-taxi drivers stated that they have ever experienced paid sex with brothel-based sex workers. Among them, approximately 30% of single military, 19.5% of single police and approximately 30% of single moto-taxi drivers have not used condoms all the time during the last three months (Sopheab et al. 1999). These figures indicate that the women workers in this study are already exposed to the risk of contracting HIV.

Women workers tended to report using condoms "all the time" in all sexual encounters, both with guests and their sweethearts. In the quantitative survey conducted as part of this study, among 42 workers who reported to have engaged in multi-partnered sex during the previous week, 27 workers stated that condoms were used in all sexual encounters. In-depth interviews conducted later, however, highlighted various constraints against condom use. Ountouch, a karaoke singer, had five regular guests last month. When she was asked whether her regular guests used condoms, she replied, "Yes. Some did. But others became very furious when I requested them to use condoms. They simply refused, and "took over my body" . . . Others were drunken, and were careless whether condoms were "on" or "off." I tried to put them on, but they refused it by force." Navin, another karaoke singer, described, "They [guests] do not want to use condoms. I persuaded them to wear condoms, but in most cases I had to put them on in order to protect the future for both of us. Some put them on by themselves reluctantly, but others shouted over me, 'If there is a virus, we will die together!' "

Serey, a beer sales promoter, had two guests three days ago, one of who was a medical staff member about 40 years old. When she requested him to wear a condom, he became angry and shouted, "I am a doctor. I don't need to use condoms!" She sighed, "He did what he wanted [sex without condoms]."

Apart from the reluctance of guests to wear condoms, the use of alcohol and drugs also increases the likelihood of unprotected sex. Takun reported that the night before she had sex with a carpenter. By the time they crawled out of the karaoke bar, both were drunk. Takun continues, "So, it was not possible to keep him still and control his behavior. He came straight into my body and ejaculated." As these narratives demonstrate, women workers explained difficulties in negotiating condom use with guests as they depend upon pleasing these guests for their economic well-being. In other cases, violence and drunkenness discourage condom use.

Women reported hardly ever using condoms with "sweethearts" or alleged cases of rape. In the above reported alleged rapes that Ountouch and other women described, no protection was used. Serey, a beer sales promoter, also reported being raped. A nephew of her stepmother wanted to marry her, but was declined by her father. One night she drank a glass of soft drink which was given by her stepmother. Suddenly, she felt dizzy and lost control of her arms and legs although she was still conscious. The nephew, Phat, entered Serey's room, and forced her to have sex. Serey claimed that it was her stepmother who set up this rape as she could then claim compensation money from Phat.

The sentiments involved in women's relationships with their regular "sweethearts" also pose a barrier to condom use. Promises of marriage as a means to court women still has persuasive power, and continues to deter condom use in the name of trust (Morris et al. 1995). Immediately after she started to work as a garment worker, Navin started to go out with a man who works as a driver in an international organization and whose parents are moneylenders in Phnom Penh. She is skeptical about the prospect of marriage, "because he is rich, and I am poor." This was confirmed after meeting his parents, who received her indifferently. Nevertheless, she loves him and he continues to promise marriage. The first time they had sex, she claimed that she suggested that he use a condom, to which he replied, "If we love each other, why do you suggest I wear condoms?" Regular sex with him, twice a week at present, has continued without condoms. He supports her every week by giving her five dollars. Likewise, Wii, a beer sales promoter, met a student in the restaurant where she works soon after she started to work in Phnom Penh. He kept on coming back to see her, said he loved her and invited her for walks. Finally, she said, "I gave my body because my sweetheart promised to take me as a future wife." In particular, the definition of a partner as a potential husband allows women to maintain sexual relationships which are defined as consistent with the prevailing discourse of appropriate femininity, *chhabap srey*. Within this discourse, Cambodian women are expected to be subordinate and obedient to their legitimate sexual partners (traditionally husbands), and respond to their sexual needs (Ledgerwood 1991). Almost all narratives which describe what workers in the sample and their sweethearts talked about, prior to their first sexual intercourse, reveal common scripts. In these scripts, men promised marriage in attempt to court women, while women begged the men to look after them or not to abandon them. There is some evidence from this study that men now play upon these cultural sexual scripts and expectations to "purchase" virginity more cheaply from female garment factory workers than from those who work at the brothels. As women "give" their bodies to men for promises of marriage and ongoing financial support, condoms are hardly ever used, despite women's fear of pregnancy and the threat of STDs and HIV/AIDS.

DISCUSSION AND CONCLUSIONS

The deepening poverty of workers' families in rural villages, and the insufficiency of their wages to support themselves in Phnom Penh, are the main determinants of women workers' entry into direct and indirect commercial sex occupations. Within the sex establishments, women report exploitative working conditions characterized by physical abuse, forced drug and alcohol intake, and exploitative wages for sexual services. These various factors combine to result in inconsistent condom use. Women's narratives also illuminate how workers differentiate between their commercial sexual partners or "guests" and their "sweethearts," which have implications for their sexual negotiations and condom use. Women view both forms of relationship as involving economic exchange, but differentiations are made on the basis of the level of emotional intimacy in the relationship, regularity and type of financial expectation.

Women garment factory workers are thus subjected to risk, structured along gradients of power. They are from poor households, with little education and are usually supporting many younger siblings. Additional vulnerability occurs when household members suffer serious illness or when there is a natural calamity. All these factors may pressure migrant daughters to participate in formal and informal sex industry occupations. As migrant factory workers, they find themselves powerless in new locations, with little social support. They work in the most repetitive jobs in the industry, receiving low wages. Within the sex industry, women workers are further subjected to violence, drug and/or alcohol use and exploitation. Those working in brothels, guesthouses and karaoke parlors experience a varying degree of vulnerability vis-à-vis sexual risks. Some brothel workers are pressured to take as many guests as possible by the proprietors who aim to optimize their profit out of women's bodies. In doing so they are at increased risk of HIV infection. Although other women in brothels and karaoke parlors report being paid per guest, they too are vulnerable as they have little discretion over who they will have sex with and limited power to negotiate with them. Workers in these two occupations are more dependent on proprietors for their economic well being than beer sales promoters or freelance sex workers, who seek and negotiate with sexual partners by themselves.

Despite the varying degree of vulnerability, particularly in terms of their negotiating power, results showed that condom use in paid sex through these occupations is inconsistent due to multiple pressures. In order to contain HIV within the core risk groups and prevent its spread to the general population, the government targets brothel-based sex workers and beer sales promoters for HIV prevention messages and condom promotion. In its most recent program initiatives, namely, 100% condom campaigns replicated from Thailand, women in these occupations (including some in the sample) are trained to persuade guests to use condoms with support provided by the brothel-owners and local police. In other words, they are expected to be the vanguards of the 100% condom campaign against HIV, a new assigned role for "virtuous" women. But these women are probably more disadvantaged than the average Cambodian woman, with low levels of education and self-esteem, subjected to multiple constraints such as violence, drug and alcohol abuse. Within a new discourse of modern virtuous women being created by the government and in some public health programs, women in these occupations are now implicitly assumed to be responsible for an increased level of consistent condom use. Empowered by education, they are expected to initiate condom use regardless of various pressures against them. In the face of this emerging expectation, denial of risks may become a dominant norm, masking the real risks.

The denial of risk occurs through the increasing definition of sexual partners as "sweethearts" rather than guests. Results show that many women reported guests as "sweethearts" as soon as a degree of communication with them, continuation or normalcy of the relationship was established. This is most pronounced among beer sales promoters who have a much longer time to socialize with and know guests before having sex than karaoke singers or brothel-based sex workers. Even brothel-based sex workers also identify regular guests as "sweethearts," a term which is not only more socially acceptable than "guests" but has implications for the nature and expectations of the relationship. In so doing, women can reorient their own identities from sex workers, a stigmatized occupation, to "virtuous" women serving men in expectation of marriage, an acceptable norm. In sexual intercourse with guests, women emphasize the externally-controlled violent action by describing guests as "tak[ing] over my body." On the other hand, in sexual intercourse with sweethearts, they emphasize their own agency: "I decided to give my body." Once male partners are identified as sweethearts, consistent condom use is even less likely. This paper shows that the risk of HIV infection needs to be understood within the structural context and relative lack of power that shape the positions of young female garment factory workers. It demonstrates the complex interrelationships between power, cultural definitions of intimacy and trust and economic security that structure sexual relationships and the risk of HIV/AIDS.

REFERENCES

Caravano, K. (1994). More than mothers and whores: redefining the AIDS prevention needs of women. In N. Krieger and R. Applemen. (eds.) *AIDS: The Politics of Survival.* Amityville, New York: Baywood.

CARE. (1998). *Meeting on Migration and HIV/AIDS in Cambodia.* Phnom Penh.

Chandler, D. (1993). *A History of Cambodia.* Second Edition. Bangkok: Silkworm.

Samrith, C. and Vonthanak, S. (1998). Report on Sentinel Surveillance in Cambodia 1998. Phnom Penh, Ministry of Health.

Farmer, P. (1999). *Infections and Inequalities: The Modern Plagues.* Berkeley: University of California Press.

Ford, N., and S Kittisuksathit. (1996a). "Mobility, love and vulnerability: sexual lifestyles of young and single factory workers in Thailand." *International Journal of Population Geography* (2), 23-33.

Ford, N., and S. Kittisuksathit. (1996b). "Youth sexuality: the sexual awareness, lifestyles and related-health service needs of young, single, factory workers in Thailand." *Nakhon Pathom, Thailand, Mahidol University, Institute for Population and Social Research [IPSR]*, 204.

Garment Manufacturers Association Cambodia. (1999). *List of Members.* Phnom Penh: Garment Manufacturers Association Cambodia.

Gorbach, P. M. (1998). *Behaviour Surveillance Survey II-1998 and Changes in Sexual Behaviour and Commercial Sex in Cambodia: 1997-1998.* Phnom Penh: National Center for HIV/AIDS, Dermatology and STDs, Ministry of Health, Cambodia.

Hall, J. A. (1999). *Human Rights and the Garment Industry in Contemporary Cambodia.* Phnom Penh: University of San Francisco.

Sopheab, H., Phalkun, M., Penh Sun, L., Someth, E., Bun Leng, H., Phalla, T., and Suwantha, S. (1999). *Cambodia's Behaviour Surveillance Survey 1999 (BSSI-III).* Phnom Penh: National Center for HIV/AIDS, Dermatology and STDs, Ministry of Health, Cambodia.

Department of Labor Inspection. (1999). *Labour Statistics: Garment Manufacturing Factories.* Phnom Penh: Department of Labor Inspection, Ministry of Social Affairs, Labour, Vocational Training and Youth Rehabilitation.

Ledgerwood, J. (1991). *Changing Khmer Conceptions of Gender: Women, Stories, and the Social Order,* Faculty of the Graduate School, Cornell University, Ithaca.

Ledgerwood, J. (1994). Gender symbolism and culture change: viewing the virtuous woman in the Khmer story "Mea Yoeng." In M. M. Ebihara, C. A. Mortland and J. Ledgerwood. (eds.) *Cambodian Culture Since 1975: Homeland and Exile.* 1994: Ithaca and London.

Ministry of Commerce. (1999). *Country Report: Cambodia.* Phnom Penh.

Morris, M., P. Anthony, P. Chai, and M. Wawer. (1995). "The relational determinants of condom use with commercial sex partners in Thailand." *AIDS* 9 (5), 507-515.

Nishigaya, K. (1999). *Poverty, Urban Migration and Risks in Urban Life, Labour Seminar: Empowerment of Women Workers.* Tokyo, Japan: Japan International Cooperation Agency.

Schoepf, B. G. (1992). Women at risk: case studies from Zaire. In G. Herdt and S. Lindenbaum. (eds.) *The Time of AIDS: Social Analysis, Theory, and Method.* Sage Publications.

Negotiating Care:
Reproductive Tract Infections in Vietnam

Maxine Whittaker, MBBS, MPH, PhD

SUMMARY. Through case studies of two women, this paper uses a taskonomy approach to analyze rural Vietnamese women's narratives of prevention, treatment and management of vaginal discharge to illustrate care seeking, health practice and the pragmatism of their action. The research is based upon ethnographic research undertaken by the author between 1995 and 1997 in a rural district in northern Vietnam. This exploration illustrates the complexities of women's rationalities and the web of influences upon their choices–the health seeking culture as practiced. The women's narratives are also placed within the broader context of gender, power and health systems that structure their decision making.

The author discusses how social and economic resource factors influence the choices women make regarding when to begin treatment for vaginal discharge and where to seek care. She concludes that women use their understanding of the relationships between health, living conditions and diseases on a day-to-day basis and that the practice of managing vaginal discharge is mediated by concepts of body, self and the body politic in Vietnam. *[Article copies available for a fee from The Haworth Document Delivery Service: 1-800-HAWORTH. E-mail address: <getinfo@ haworthpressinc.com> Website: <http://www.HaworthPress.com> © 2002 by The Haworth Press, Inc. All rights reserved.]*

Maxine Whittaker is Senior Lecturer, Australian Centre for International Health and Nutrition, The University of Queensland, and Deputy Team Leader, Health Services Support Program, National Department of Health, P.O. Box 1182, Waigani NCD, Papua New Guinea (E-mail: mwhittaker@hssp.com.pg).

[Haworth co-indexing entry note]: "Negotiating Care: Reproductive Tract Infections in Vietnam." Whittaker, Maxine. Co-published simultaneously in *Women & Health* (The Haworth Medical Press, an imprint of The Haworth Press, Inc.) Vol. 35, No. 4, 2002, pp. 43-57; and: *Women's Health in Mainland Southeast Asia* (ed: Andrea Whittaker) The Haworth Medical Press, an imprint of The Haworth Press, Inc., 2002, pp. 43-57. Single or multiple copies of this article are available for a fee from The Haworth Document Delivery Service [1-800-HAWORTH, 9:00 a.m. - 5:00 p.m. (EST). E-mail address: getinfo@haworthpressinc. com].

43

KEYWORDS. Reproductive tract infections, Vietnam, qualitative methods, care-seeking behavior

INTRODUCTION

In Vietnam, when women suffer from a health problem, they make decisions about when, where, from whom and how much care to seek within a pluralistic health system. Traditional practices based on *Thuoc bac* (Northern medicine, derived from Chinese traditional medicine) and *Thuoc nam* (Southern medicine, traditional Vietnamese medicine) are widely used through growing or collecting one's own herbs and foods, or through markets or traditional practitioners. Western medical care, including pharmaceuticals, is obtained through pharmacies, the government sector and the private sector. In this paper, I analyze rural Vietnamese women's narratives of prevention, treatment and management of vaginal discharge to illustrate care seeking, health practice and the pragmatism of their actions.

The data used was collected during ethnographic fieldwork between 1995 and 1997 in a rural district in northern Vietnam. I combined 67 participant observations, 37 focus group and 72 in-depth interviews with free listing, pile sorting and content analysis in an iterative process. Between 1997 and 1998, feedback to the community, providers and policy makers informed the analysis. From this work, I sought to develop a taxonomy for vaginal discharge, which revealed the denotative features of vaginal discharge. Pile sorting illustrated how these names could be organized into units referring to color, smell, seriousness, and prevalence. However, these units and their relationships often were inconsistent across and among groups of women, and did not easily or clearly link to biomedical classifications (Zurayk et al. 1995; Gorbach et al. 1998; see also Boonmongkon et al. this issue). There is a flexible interrelationship between perceived etiologies, life circumstances and, as explored below, tasks or actions women take. Incongruities and irrationalities in the actions and decisions taken by women may emerge. Hunt and Mattingly (1998:268) call these "divergent rationalities" that affect the sufferer and the healers, "a multiple form of reasoning simultaneously providing multiple visions, multiple versions of the illness and thus multiple guides to appropriate action."

The "taskonomy" approach to seeking and using care focuses on everyday behavior of people where they recognize and act upon distinctions of some sort in the symptoms or illness experience (Dougherty and Keller 1982; Nichter and Nichter 1996). The strategies women take are oriented particularly to their social, cultural, and economic circumstances, and characteristics of the illness being experienced at the time. This pragmatic organization of behavior has an end in mind–relief of symptoms that are worrisome, or prevention of a serious manifestation of the illness, whilst limiting social and economic costs. These organizations of behavior may vary according to the circumstances when they next have the symptoms. Women cannot always be "a rational actor, promoted by self interest" (Hunt and Mattingly 1998:267), with an ability to access and consider a range of options to help her best attain her goals. If the analysis of a woman's behavior is limited to "conceptualising practical reasoning solely within a framework of instrumental logic, one misses much of the everyday thinking that occurs when people confront illness" (Hunt and Mattingly 1998:267). A taskonomy approach takes into account other experiences in a woman's life influencing her decisions.

In this paper, I examine health seeking culture as practiced through the detailed case studies of two women, Binh and Dung. Vietnamese women's decision making is not related simply to means-and-ends mapped taxonomically. Rather, decision making is fluid, contextual and opportunistic, informed by women's own experiences and those of their families and peers. Individual cases illustrate the complex relationships between lived experiences, social and economic realities, power and the significance of these relationships for the women involved (Good 1994).

CASE STUDY 1: BINH

I met Binh, a 40-year-old Catholic woman and mother of 5 children, during my first week in the commune. With 20 other women, she was waiting at the commune health station for the "weekly" mobile team visit. Sitting in the crowded waiting area, Binh told me that she wanted another IUD inserted because she did not want any more children after this "last boy," a "mistake" caused by the IUD slipping out, 14 years after the birth of her last son. Giang, my research assistant, and I arranged to meet her later that week in her home. Over several weeks, we met and talked with her and her family, sharing meals, jokes and stories. On one occasion, we were discussing women's experiences with vaginal discharge and her reactions to it.

If one is hot inside, the discharge is *huyet xau*. If you are hot inside you must drink *thuoc mat*. It is a refreshing medicine to prevent you developing an infection . . . So you have to find fresh things to cool you–like lemon, sugar, fresh leaves. Fresh leaves like *nho noi, la rau ma, co muc, rau sam* . . . They are easy to find here on the streets and on the grass banks. *Nha nei* and *rau ma* are *thuec nam* (Southern medicine). You could also use *la chuoi chap* and *la me giai*, but we don't have these here . . . Also *la phuong vu* and *cu can truat*. You pound the leaves to have the juice and then add sugar and drink it. You drink this and wash in *la oi* as a complementary treatment. These are the medicines for infection (*thuoc viem*). Nowadays many women take Western medicines–but they are hot. So if you take *thuoc tay* (Western medicine), you have to find fresh things to eat . . . If the discharge or the infection is too serious, you have to go to the district hospital to have it washed . . . The leaves only wash and clean the bacteria. Or the same if you use salt. It sterilizes but it does not kill the bacteria. So washing makes you hygienic. But if you have disease, you must have medicine. These have the effect of killing the bacteria, so you use them for infections. The leaves you boil like *la oi, sim, tra xanh* are for washing . . .

Sometimes I have an infection with itch and *lo lo mau ca* (fish blood). This is very harmful . . . It is so itchy that I want to put a finger inside and hook it out. I scratch and scratch. Many women have the same and want to do the same. I wash with salt water and take *ampi* (ampicillin). Then it is relieved and it gets better. Some women are lazy and don't want to take medicines. Then it gets serious and the discharge is like red blood. When you wash you see red blood.

Another time as we sat on the dirt floor of her home during a lunch break from transplanting, Binh told us of her war-invalid husband's health problems–he had been crying in pain all night, unable to get relief. This pain was a recurrent problem for him and meant he could not work. It exacerbated their poverty. Like their neighbors, they believe the poor quality low-lying land is allocated to them because they are Catholic. They lost the second rice crop last year and are very short of money. Her 17-year-old daughter is working as hired labor on a farm 2 hours' walk from home. Binh had been working hard all day, with little sleep and little food to eat. She was concerned about the effect this would have on her health, particularly her reproductive health.

> When I have a bad period, the blood is black. It is like the color of the water from boiling sweet potato leaves (*nuoc rau lang*) . . . It is bad. Some women take medicine . . . The medicine they take is one that you buy from the practitioner . . . His name is *Ong Vinh*. He has *thuoc hoan tan* pills. Or you can buy this medicine from a shop in the market. It is a powdery medicine, mixed with honey and sugar and rolled into a pill . . . But I don't have the money for this medicine . . . Usually you need to take 4-5 pills, 2 times a day . . . It is because I work hard and eat little that I have this discharge problem. This year we lost our paddy crop. I had to earn money by going to the forest to collect wood. I had to carry a heavy load–30 to 40 kilograms for 8-9 kilometers from the forest. Carrying a heavy load is harmful for the menstruation.

Binh's complex narratives demonstrate the pluralistic nature of the knowledge used to make sense of vaginal discharge. Humoral concepts, social and moral discourses, her role as a mother, and economic hardship are all entailed in her description of her health.

As Binh explains, some discharges are due to being hot inside the body and others may be due to bacteria. She also links these humoral concepts with ethnophysiological understandings of blood, and links between 'bad' blood and menstrual problems (Gammeltoft 1999; see also Boonmongkon et al. this volume). This distinction guides her choice of appropriate treatment. Hot conditions should be treated with something cooling. In describing cooling medicines, she demonstrates an understanding of a range of traditional herbal treatments that could be used (Craig 1997). Many of these grow near the home, and so are easily accessible.

She also expresses concerns about the "hotness" of Western medicines. In Vietnam many people discuss how Western medicines are fast acting, but strong and hot, whereas traditional medicines are slower, but neutral or cooling (Craig 1997; Gammeltoft 1999). Beliefs that antibiotics are hot affect their use in Vietnam. Antibiotics need some adjuvant to cool the body (to prevent other health problems). Vitamin C and Vitamin B1 are commonly requested for this purpose. Additionally the user may limit the duration of use of these antibiotics to a sub-optimal or non-therapeutic level (Halfvarson et al. 1995), increasing chances of antibiotic resistant bacteria developing (Phuong Dinh Thu 1997).

The perceived aetiology will also affect treatment. If the aetiology of the illness is believed to be "traditionally" based, then traditional care is more likely to be sought. For example, a perceived imbalance between the binary forces of hot/cold, or *am/duong* (the Vietnamese equivalent to the Chinese concept of yin/yang), will encourage patients to seek restoration of balance either as the sole treatment or as part of the treatment regime. If Western or other medicines have proven effective and suitable to the client for this illness in previous experiences, they may be used again.

Concern about the seriousness of the discharge triggers a decision for Binh to seek some treatment other than traditional medicines or hygienic behaviors. Women describe changes in color, smell, or profuseness of the discharge, presence of a fever, and the linkage with severe abdominal pain as markers of a change from "light" to "heavy" disease. The symptoms and signs of RTIs in women are subtle and more difficult to diagnose than in men (Dallabetta et al. 1998). Often they may be similar to normal physiological events such as some vaginal discharges (Dadian 1996). Additionally many women may not know of their risk. Their sexual partner may not discuss their illness with them because it is embarrassing or may raise questions about fidelity, trust and blame (Steen 1996). In many settings, including in Vietnam, women believe themselves not at risk of sexually transmitted diseases or HIV due to their personal monogamy (Tran Hung Minh et al. 1999; Brugemann and Franklin 1997). Vietnamese women and their providers do not perceive rural men as having the time or energy (because of hard work) to be anything but monogamous (Whittaker, M. 2000). Many women wait until there is an exacerbation of their symptoms before they "self-identify" as being ill with an RTI. This may result in a more complex presentation of their illness.

Previous studies in Vietnam identified the distinction between "light" and "heavy" illness and the ability to afford treatment as major decision points (Craig 1997). But other variables affect women's decisions to seek "higher" level care, especially those that require money. One of these variables is if the illness or symptoms interfere with her ability to work (becoming too uncomfortable or inconvenient). Another consideration is the woman's ability to maintain sexual relationships with her husband (because it is painful, may worsen the condition or may be transmitted). A third variable is if the perceived consequences of leaving it untreated are serious, even life threatening (such as turning into gonorrhea or syphilis, cancer or infertility).

Binh's case also reflects the predominance in women's, providers' and government narratives of discharge being linked to poor hygiene– being "dirty" (see Boonmongkon et al. this volume). Women like Binh use hygienic washing as the major first line of action. Providers pre- scribe washing as part of the treatment regime. The health care staff dis- courses often elaborate upon the role of bacteria as the main cause of the discharge, neglecting other potential causes of discharge unrelated to hygiene or bacteria. Because of this predominance of a bacterial aetiol- ogy in women's and providers' narratives, including in health education materials and in diagnosis, the resort to antibiotic use to "kill" bacteria is a common and dominant practice.

The ability to afford treatment, traditional or Western, is an impor- tant factor in choice of care. Binh's discussions illustrate the dou- ble-edged sword of poverty, from her and her peers' perspectives. Because they are poor, they must do things that are harmful to their health, like carrying heavy loads. And because they are poor, they can- not afford to treat the problems that are caused by hard work. Her vivid description of the extremes of discomfort that some women bear before seeking care are linked to ability to pay and perceived seriousness of the conditions.

In some ways, like many other women, Binh blames herself for the dysmenorrhea and bad periods and other discharge problems. She can- not rest when she should, cannot eat "strengthening up" foods to restore her blood, and cannot follow instructions regarding post-IUD insertion behavior. This also makes her reluctant to seek further care–because she may have, in some way or degree, caused the problem.

CASE 2: DUNG

Dung was a 28-year-old woman I met by the roadside one morning, looking at her paddy fields. She was deciding whether to prepare the fields that day, or stay home with her 4-year-old daughter and her 18-month-old son, who she was still complementary breast-feeding. She was urged by her in-laws to continue to breast feed her son so he will be strong and healthy. Similar behaviour was not supported for her daughter, who Dung now worries is a bit small and weakly. Although her 76-year-old mother lives with her and can look after the children, Dung would rather be at home. We walked past the fruit trees she had growing, up three steps into the cement-floored, three-roomed house.

As we drank green tea and played with her children, she discussed her first experiences with vaginal discharge.

> The time when I had an itch, I wondered what was the matter with me. I had heard that having an itch may mean that you have an infection. I was worried. So I asked a woman who had had an itch and was examined at the commune health station. She told me about the female hygienic washing powders. I bought some from the health station and I read the packet and then used them for a few days. And it went away. So now I always use them everyday . . . to keep clean and prevent it . . . and use them more during the menstrual time . . . I just use it to wash. I have heard that infected people have to sit in it.

Itch is often the precursor of a discharge according to the women interviewed. In this discussion, Dung describes a fairly typical approach to care when a women experiences a symptom like itch or discharge for the first time. She was concerned about this new symptom, which occurred reasonably early in her married life, and did not know what it really meant. Many women discussed how they thought vaginal discharge and other gynecological problems, except bad periods, were predominantly a problem for women after they become sexually active. Women hear little from parents or relatives before marriage about sexual health or sexuality (Le Thi Nham Tuyet et al. 1993; Khuat Thu Hong 1998). The occurrence of a symptom like itch, discharge or, as some women discuss, painful urination, makes them concerned.

Dung was concerned that she may have an infection which was potentially serious and needed treatment. She sought advice from other women who had learnt through their own experience. This demonstrates the networking that occurs among women, sharing some details of their gynecological experiences, even though many state that it is still shameful or embarrassing to talk about these sorts of things. Women learn from their own experiences, and from each other, about actions to take when they have various symptoms such as the use of female hygiene washing powders bought over the counter at the commune health station. Dung, with such advice in hand, and an ability to read, as can the majority of women in the Red River Delta Region, saw no need for further assistance. She used the powders according to instructions on the packet (none were given when she bought them), and the symptoms resolved.

Dung's discussions also demonstrate the concern about hygiene and uncleanliness being the cause of such symptoms. Some of this concern may be well founded. Smegma, vaginal secretions and environmental conditions, as well as fecal material, play a role, if left uncleaned, in causing local genital itch, inflammation and infections. However it goes beyond that. Female washing powders are thought by women and providers to sterilize the water, making it, and the areas washed, cleaner. The need for increased attention to hygiene during menstruation is understood to refer not only to being physically clean. It also refers to the issues of menstrual blood being dirty and menstruation being a time when bacteria can more readily enter the women's reproductive organs. Government and health messages reinforce this need for increased attention to hygiene during menstruation, recommending washing three times a day and changing clothes at lunchtime. In addition, there is a belief that soaking in water allows the inside of the woman's organs to be cleaned, just as soaking in paddy field water increases a woman's chance of bad air and bacteria getting inside.

Dung's husband doesn't live with her. He works in the neighboring district in a middle management job. He is now closer than before, and she is worried that "self-family planning" (withdrawal, calendar methods and/or periodic abstinence) is no longer adequate protection against pregnancy. He visits more often now, sometimes unexpectedly on his motorbike. She was thinking about using an IUD again. Her last experience with vaginal discharge was related to an abortion. She had delayed having the abortion for two weeks until her husband had come home. The delay meant the abortion cost more money due to the later gestational age, and she was "scolded" by the providers for coming late.

> I had an abortion in August at the district hospital . . . After the abortion I rested for about 30 minutes and then returned home. . . When I came home I had some more rest. On this day my husband cooked the meals–just normal foods and eggs and fruit. The hospital gave me 10 tablets of *ampi* (ampicillin) . . . I am not sure what they were for, maybe to avoid infection. After the abortion when I got off the table I felt a little dizzy. I came home and I had some abdominal pain and felt uncomfortable. This lasted only 3-4 days . . . When I had the pain some liquid came out. My husband crushed some *rau ngot* and gave it to me with some water to drink . . . After I drank the *rau ngot* I had no more abdominal pain, but a lot of liquid came out for 2 days and it was prolonged for almost a week . . . When it was a lot it came out *huyet do* (red blood). Sometimes it

came out *nhay nhay* (very sticky), *trang trang* (very white), *lo lo* (colored) . . . they call it *lo lo mau ca* (color of fish blood) . . . The next week *lo lo trang trang* (discharge colored very white) came out a little and very sticky. But I didn't do anything about it–only talked with my husband . . . The day not much came out but I had pain my husband said it was like something was stuck, and that made the pain in my abdomen. He gave me the *rau ngot* water to drink and it came out. So I had very little pain.

Her case illustrates the practice amongst Vietnamese providers to provide ampicillin (to avoid infection), vitamin C (to cool the body) and papaverine (mistakenly used to reduce uterine contractions) to women after menstrual regulations, abortions and IUD insertions. As discussed earlier, the prescribing of antibiotics reinforces in women's and providers' minds the link between these three procedures and vaginal discharge and infections. But it can also be a source of anxiety for women. Many women discussed how they knew that not taking their medicines after an IUD insertion or abortion was a cause of vaginal discharge. But they also saw the 20 tablets of ampicillin as a useful resource for the household for childhood infections. Many women take only a few or none of the ampicillin, storing it instead for potential future use by their children, when ill. But doing so makes them feel responsible for any consequent discharge. Thus they avoid seeking care from the health care provider and self treat to avoid being scolded for not following instructions.

From her peers' point of view, Dung is fortunate to have a husband with such empathy for his wife. He helped her prevent the problem becoming more serious by providing her the opportunity to have treatment and eat well after the procedure. Women talked about the need to inform their husbands about the management of vaginal discharge, abortions or commencing use of a contraceptive (Johansson et al. 1998). For most women in Vietnam, this is not strictly to seek permission. However, this means that their husbands have been informed, so that if financial, "emotional" or other resources are required to manage the vaginal discharge or recuperate after the abortion or manage contraceptive side effects, they will be available (Nichter 1992).

Dung described her specific management for a specific cause of discharge–post-abortion discharge. The narrative illustrates the multiple terms women use to describe discharges and their characteristics. Dung's husband had some knowledge of traditional medical theories and treatments, such as the concept of something causing a blockage and requiring a medicine, *rau ngot*, that is bitter and cold (Reid 1987) and able to reduce the swelling. His knowledge of treatment and its success in resolving her problem meant that she did not seek further treatment nor advice. She stated that she only had "normal" food, but eggs and fruit is not part of the normal diet in this commune or this household. The fruit is also cooling, and depending on which type, may be bitter, enhancing the effect from the herbal medicines. Eggs are a strengthening food to help restore health after an abortion or other weakening events. Dung's statement may reflect that she felt these were normal foods in such circumstances or that dietary aspects of maintaining health are so normalized in everyday life that there is nothing "special" about it. Dung's case illustrates the ways in which families and households are involved in maintaining, seeking and restoring health of family members (Berman, et al. 1994).

One of the reasons why Dung, who had attained her desired family size (2 children), did not speak to others about her discharge, even with family, was that she had an abortion. She described the disapproval she would face had her parents-in-law or other relatives heard that she had an abortion. Dung was living the Vietnamese family planning ideal of a two-child family, and had internalized messages of giving children a better education, better life, happiness and health if there were only two. But many people express anxiety about abortion (Gammeltoft and Nguyen Minh Thang 1999; Johansson et al. 1998). Traditionally, abortion was thought to be a sin after 12-14 weeks, when the fetus is no longer just a blood clot, but looks like a frog (Gammeltoft 1999; see also Whittaker A. this issue). It is possible that Dung's in-laws held this value. The possibility of having another son was also important for the lineage of the family within Confucian values. Others in the community may think her ignorant and backward for becoming pregnant, given the societal value placed on control and a two-child family.

Women, men and providers also perceive that abortions drain a women's health and vitality similar to childbirth (Gammeltoft 1999). If a woman is young, healthy and could "afford" the State fines for having a third child, her in-laws and others may not understand why she would seek to have an abortion rather than a child. This disapproval limited Dung's options of care. In keeping the decision to herself and her husband, she was able to avoid a variety of social costs.

DISCUSSION

Women's treatment and care decisions are not made purely on the basis of a taxonomic classification of disease and symptoms. Their vaginal discharge illness narratives "reveal the practices and ideologies that encode structures of social relations and power, as these shape the rhythms of illness and therapy" (Good 1994:134).

Most models of health behaviour attempt to predict decision making as linear, to identify ways of influencing behaviors and to measure the success of those interventions. Most of these behavior theories take an etic, deductive approach, testing their ideas of what influences the behaviour of seeking and using health care to produce predictive models of behavior (Becker 1974; Fishbein et al. 1991; Hornik 1991). These behavioral models of health seeking have been, and remain, highly influential in health promotion and social marketing programs in health. However, they are inadequate. They remove everyday realities of a person's life from the model. These models assume that a person's life is constant, and value cognitive processes of weighing risk, susceptibility, benefits and barriers more highly than that of the daily tasks of living and the need to fit health decision making into this reality. "People who fall ill must choose between multiple and competing systems of healing" (Brodwin 1996:13) and may combine elements from diverse or even contradictory medical traditions in their help seeking activities (Whittaker, A. 2000).

I show how Vietnamese women's concerns to continue to work, maintain family harmony and contribute financially to the family are important considerations in their choices. The women with whom I spoke were not always "free to decide and free to act." Body politics, gender relationships, health care management and economics, and social norms of cleanliness, family life and the boundaries of acceptable behaviour all influence their decisions and actions. Additionally, the woman's understanding of why she is experiencing the vaginal discharge influences her decisions of when to act, what actions to take and how long to pursue the action.

A taskonomy of vaginal discharge demonstrates how women use their understanding of relationships between health, living conditions and diseases on a day-to-day basis. This emic based approach of how vaginal discharge is managed and negotiated in women's family and social lives assists in identifying variables that influence choices (Garro 1998). These may be points for programmatic intervention to enable women improve their lives and health. Vietnamese health programs' focus upon training providers on the syndromic approach to reproductive tract infection management and providing health education messages to women about washing themselves are missing the needs of women. Women need improved knowledge of their bodies, increased access and affordability of appropriate care, as well as access to clean and safe water and sanitation.

Various decision points and resorts to treatment operate for vaginal discharge as discussed in the case studies. However, there are problems in trying to represent decision making as a purely rational process. Multiple forms of reasoning occur with every episode of vaginal discharge. These may vary with time, experience, seasons, and mood (Brodwin 1996). Examining "particular instances when care seekers or their healers struggle to deal with serious illness" (Hunt and Mattingly 1998:268) allows one to comprehend the divergent rationalities that are involved in reasoning for care seeking in the management of vaginal discharge. It also illustrates the various co-existing and sometimes conflicting discourses and "visions" of the affliction of vaginal discharge and its management that affect the choice of management. The notions of vaginal discharge and its management are not a stable cultural system, but are embedded in "the informal logic of everyday life, animated through specific healing activities and articulated with overarching material and ideological forces" (Brodwin 1996:15-16). The practice of managing vaginal discharge is mediated by concepts of body, self, and the body politic in Vietnam, especially regarding women's bodies and reproduction from the family, religion and political systems.

REFERENCES

Becker, M. (1974). The health belief model and sick role behavior. *Health Education Monographs* 2: 409-419.

Berman, P., C. Kendall, and K. Bhattacharyya (1994). The household production of health: integrating social science perspectives on micro-level health determinants. *Social Science and Medicine* 38(2): 205-215.

Brodwin, P. (1996). *Medicine and Morality in Haiti: The Contest of Healing Power.* Cambridge: Cambridge University Press.

Brugemann, I. and B. Franklin (1997). *Love and the Risk of AIDS for Women in Vietnam.* Ha Noi: CARE International in Vietnam.

Craig, D. A. (1997). Familiar Medicine: Local and Global Health and Development in Vietnam. Unpublished PhD thesis. Canberra: Department of Human Geography, The Australian National University.

Dadian, M. J. (1996). Syndromic management : promoting effective STD diagnosis in resource-poor settings. *AIDScaptions* May: 9-13.

Dallabetta, G., A. Gerbase, and K. Holmes (1998). Problems, solutions and challenges in syndromic management of sexually transmitted diseases. *Sexually Transmitted Infections* 74 (Suppl 1): S1-S11.

Do Trong Hieu, Pham Thuy Nga, Nguyen Kim Tong, Vu Quy Nhan, Nguyen Thi Thom et al. (1995). *An Assessment of the Need for Contraceptive Introduction in Vietnam.* Geneva: WHO.

Do Trong Hieu and J. Stoeckel (1993). Pregnancy termination and contraceptive failure in Vietnam. *Asia Pacific Population Journal* 8(4): 3-18.

Dougherty, J. W. and C. M. Keller (1982). Taskonomy: a practical approach to knowledge structures. *American Ethnologist* 9(4): 763-774.

Fishbein, M., S. E. Middlestadt, and P. Hitchcock (1991). Using information to change sexually transmitted disease-related behaviors: an analysis based on the Theory of Reasoned Action. In J. N. Wasserheit, S. O. Aral, K. K. Holmes and P. J. Hitchcock (eds.) *Research Issues in Human Behaviour and Sexually Transmitted Diseases in the AIDS Era.* Washington DC: American Society for Microbiology, 243-257.

Gammeltoft, T. M. (1999). *Women's Bodies, Women's Worries: Health and Family Planning in a Vietnamese Rural Community.* Richmond: Curzon Press.

Gammeltoft, T. M. and Nguyen Minh Thang (1999). *Our Love Has no Limits.* Ha Noi, Nha Xuat Ban Thanh Nien.

Garro, L. C. (1998). On the rationality of decision making studies: Part 1: Decision models of treatment choice. *Medical Anthropology Quarterly* 11(2): 319-340.

Good, B. (1994). *Medicine, Rationality and Experience: An Anthropological Perspective.* Cambridge, Cambridge University Press.

Gorbach, P., Dao T. Khanh Hoa, A. Tsui, and Vu Quy Nhan (1998). Reproduction, Risk and Reality: Family Planning and Reproductive Health in Northern Vietnam. *Journal of Biosocial Sciences* 30: 393-409.

Halfvarson, J., N. Heijne et al. (1995). Rural mother's perceptions of antibiotics in their use against ARI among children five years and under in the Uong Bi district, Quang Ninh, Vietnam. Report. Stockholm: Karolinska Institute.

Hornik, R. (1991). Alternative models of behaviour change. In J. N. Wasserheit, S. O. Aral, K. K. Holmes and P. J. Hitchcock (eds.) *Research Issues in Human Behaviour and Sexually Transmitted Diseases in the AIDS Era.* (pp. 201-218). Washington DC: American Society for Microbiology.

Hunt, L. M. and C. Mattingly (1998). Diverse rationalities and multiple realities in illness and healing. *Medical Anthropology Quarterly* 12(3): 267-272.

Johansson, A. (1998). *Dreams and Dilemmas–Women and Family Planning in Rural Vietnam.* Stockholm, Karolinska Institute.

Johansson, A., Nguyen Thu Nga, Tran Quang Huy, Doan Du Dat, and K. Holmgren (1998). Husband's involvement in abortion in Vietnam. *Studies in Family Planning* 29(4): 1-14.

Johansson, A., Hoang Thi Hoa, Le Thi Nham Tuyet, Mai Bich, and B. Hojer (1996). Family planning in Vietnam–women's experiences and dilemma: a community study from the Red River Delta. *Journal of Psychosomatic Obstetrics and Gynecology* 17: 59-67.

Khuat Thu Hong (1998). Study on Sexuality in Vietnam: The Known and Unknown Factors. *Regional Working Papers–South and East Asia: The Population Council.* Ha Noi: The Population Council.

Le Thi Nham Tuyet, Nguyen The Lap, and Hoang Thi Hoa (1993). Summary Report on Sexual and Reproduction Health of Adolescents in Some Provinces in Vietnam. Unpublished report, Ha Noi: Center for Women's Research and Teaching.

Nichter, M. (1992). Health social science research on the study of diarrhoeal disease: a focus on dysentery. In M. Nichter and M. Nichter (eds.) *Anthropology and International Health. Asian Case Studies.* (pp. 111-134) Amsterdam: Gordon and Breach Publishers.

Nichter, M. and M. Nichter (1996). *Anthropology and International Health: Asian Case Studies.* Amsterdam: Gordon and Breach Publishers.

Phuong Dinh Thu (1997). Towards rational use of antibiotics in Vietnam: present status of infectious diseases in Vietnam. *Australian Prescriber* 20 (Suppl 1): 134-136.

Reid, D. (1987). *Chinese Herbal Medicines.* Hong Kong: CFW Publications.

Steen, R. (1996). Studies show partner notification contributes to STD control. *AIDScaptions* (May): 28-30.

Tran Hung Minh, Vu Song Ha, and Hoang Tu Anh (1999). *RTI: Current Situation of the Diseases. The Gaps of Knowledge and Practice of Women of Child Bearing Age in a Rural Area of Vietnam.* Ha Noi: Medical Publishing House.

Whittaker, A. (2000). *Intimate Knowledge: Women and Their Health in North-East Thailand.* St Leonards: Allen and Unwin.

Whittaker, M. (2000). *Secret Stories: Women's Health in Rural Vietnam.* Unpublished PhD Thesis, Brisbane: Tropical Health Program, University of Queensland.

Zurayk, H., H. Khattab, N. Younis, O. Kamal, and M. El-Helw (1995). Comparing women's reports with medical diagnoses of reproductive tract morbidity conditions in rural Egypt. *Studies in Family Planning* 26:14-21.

Women's Health in Northeast Thailand: Working at the Interface Between the Local and the Global

Pimpawun Boonmongkon, PhD
Mark Nichter, PhD
Jen Pylypa, MA
Niporn Sanhajariya, MA
Soiboon Saitong, MA

Pimpawun Boonmongkon is Associate Professor of Medical Anthropology and Acting Director, Niporn Sanhajariya and Soiboon Saitong are Researchers at the Center for Health Policy Studies, Faculty of Health Social Science & Humanities, Mahidol University, Salaya Campus, 25/25 Phutthamonthon Road 4, Salaya, Nakhon Pathom 73170, Thailand. Mark Nichter is Professor of Medical Anthropology, and Jen Pylypa is a PhD candidate, Department of Anthropology, Emil W. Haury Building, University of Arizona, Tucson, AZ 85721 USA.

Address correspondence to: Mark Nichter, Department of Anthropology, Emil W. Haury Building, University of Arizona, Tucson, AZ 85721 USA (E-mail: mnichter@ u.arizona.edu).

This collaborative study was conducted with the assistance of staff from the Center for Health Policy Studies, Mahidol University, and the Faculty of Pharmacy and the Faculty of Nursing, Khon Kaen University. The authors offer special thanks to project consultants Dr. Christopher Elias of the Population Council, Thailand, and Dr. Suwanna Warakamin, Director of the Family Health and Population Division, Ministry of Health, Thailand. The authors would also like to express their sincere thanks to all the women, health volunteers, and health staff in Khon Kaen Province who gave their time and shared their experiences in order to make this research possible.

Funding for this project was provided by the Ford Foundation, Thailand and Vietnam. A sabbatical grant from the Rockefeller Foundation (1997-98) enabled Dr. Nichter's full participation.

[Haworth co-indexing entry note]: "Women's Health in Northeast Thailand: Working at the Interface Between the Local and the Global." Boonmongkon, Pimpawun et al. Co-published simultaneously in *Women & Health* (The Haworth Medical Press, an imprint of The Haworth Press, Inc.) Vol. 35, No. 4, 2002, pp. 59-80; and: *Women's Health in Mainland Southeast Asia* (ed: Andrea Whittaker) The Haworth Medical Press, an imprint of The Haworth Press, Inc., 2002, pp. 59-80. Single or multiple copies of this article are available for a fee from The Haworth Document Delivery Service [1-800-HAWORTH, 9:00 a.m. - 5:00 p.m. (EST). E-mail address: getinfo@haworthpressinc.com].

SUMMARY. An important first step in translating global statements about women's right to health into action programs is an assessment of the interface between local health culture and public health/medical practice. In this paper, we present the findings of an ongoing research project focusing on women's sexual and reproductive health in Northeast Thailand. The project is a prototype illustrating how formative research may be used to guide intervention development as well as midcourse correction. Examples are provided which clearly illustrate why cultural understandings of gynecological health are important to consider before introducing women's health programs. One case featured describes how an iatrogenic fear of cervical cancer has emerged from public health messages and screening programs. A hybrid model of cancer has evolved from preexisting local ideas, resulting in an exaggerated sense of risk wherein women fear that a wide range of common problems may potentially transform into this fatal disease. We argue that public health needs to be held accountable for what transpires when health messages are introduced into a community. Monitoring of community response is necessary. In the second half of the paper we describe efforts to increase community understanding of women's health problems, create gender and culturally sensitive health care services, and enhance the technical and communication skills of health staff. *[Article copies available for a fee from The Haworth Document Delivery Service: 1-800-HAWORTH. E-mail address: <getinfo@haworthpressinc.com> Website: <http://www.HaworthPress.com> © 2002 by The Haworth Press, Inc. All rights reserved.]*

KEYWORDS. Women's health, gynecology, reproductive health, Thailand, gender-sensitivity, cultural-sensitivity

Over the past decade, increasing international attention has been focused on women's sexual and reproductive health as a priority area for health care reform. New women's health agenda and "global right to health" discourses emerged out of the Programme of Action of the International Population and Development Conference held in Cairo in 1994, and the Beijing Platform for Action Conference held in 1997 (DeJong 2000; Hempel 1996). Women's health advocates argued that heath care reform required a careful consideration of women's experiences of sexual as well as reproductive health, the accessibility and quality of health care available to women, and cultural and gender dimensions of health that impact women's sense of vulnerability and perceptions of well being. Following these conferences, women's health advocates have been faced with the difficult challenges of (1) lobbying for actual changes in health policy agreed upon in principle by high ranking government officials, (2) finding ways to implement new policy changes in institutional environments where local health care providers have been socialized to respond to a limited set of public health indicators (Hardee et al. 1999; WHO 1999), (3) retraining health staff to be more gender and culturally sensitive to women's health problems, and (4) teaching women how to better manage common health problems, access health services, and present their problems to health care providers.

An important first step in translating global statements about women's right to health into action programs has been an assessment of the interface between local health culture and public health/medical practice. Several studies have found that there is dissonance between local perceptions of reproductive health and women's self-reports of illness on the one hand, and rates of reproductive morbidity documented by epidemiological studies on the other (see Sadana 2000 for an overview). A balanced approach to women's health problems has been called for which pays as much attention to women's social and cultural experiences of reproductive health as to the presence or absence of identifiable disease. In order to implement health care reform, there is a need to get beyond both narrow visions of evidence-based medicine that discount the experiences of women (Boonmongkon et al. 2001), and general discussions of women's rights to health which deflect attention away from the range of women's experiences and the specific factors influencing those experiences.

In this paper, we present the findings of an ongoing formative research project focusing on women's sexual and reproductive health in Northeast Thailand. Our use of the term "formative research" (Boonmongkon et al. 1998) refers to a grounded investigation of popular health culture, health care seeking behavior, and health care provision as a means of informing critical thinking about health care reform. Two stages of the project will be discussed: an initial, informative research stage and an intervention development stage. During both stages of the project, the research team was attentive to the impact of global flows of knowledge as they influenced both those being "studied" in local health care arenas (community members and health care providers) and those conducting formative research. Drawing upon Ginsburg and Rapp (1995), we use the term *global* to refer to knowledge and power which flows beyond the communities of its creation to be embraced by or imposed on others. Applied to the study of women's health, the global encompasses discourses about women generated by public health and medical experts who speak through the "universal" language of science, and the discourses of women's health advocates who speak for all women using the language of social justice and universal rights. The *local* denotes any small-scale arena in which social meanings are informed and adjusted through negotiated, face-to-face interactions. Within local health arenas, longstanding and newly introduced, global health conceptualizations, discourses, and practices converge, resulting in juxtaposition, appropriation and hybridization.

STAGE ONE: ETHNOGRAPHIC RESEARCH

The initial stage of formative research was carried out in 1997 in three rural districts of Khon Kaen Province, Northeast Thailand, an ethnic Lao (Isan) rice-growing region of the country. The project involved a multidisciplinary team composed of medical anthropologists, doctors, nurses, pharmacists, and women's health advocates. The research objectives were to document women's experiences and understandings of gynecological complaints and their related self-care and health care seeking patterns, to assess local government health services available to women, and to generate ideas for promising lines of intervention.

Data collection involved a variety of research methods, only some of which will be mentioned here.[1] Research began with a community-based survey administered to 1028 women of reproductive age in sixteen villages across three districts of Khon Kaen Province. The survey yielded data on self-reported prevalence of women's problems (over the past two weeks, two months, and two years), Pap smear clinic attendance, self-medication, and the utilization of health services for women's problems. Following the survey, an intensive ethnographic study was conducted over two months, employing participant-observation as well as structured and semi-structured interviews and focus groups. Ethnographic research aimed to document women's experiences of "gynecological complaints," a term we use broadly to encompass (1) symptoms commonly associated with reproductive tract infections, and (2) pelvic, lower abdominal and back pains associated with hard manual labor, childbearing, menstruation, etc., as well as other symptoms linked to the "uterus" (*mot luk*) through cultural reasoning. Data were collected on notions of ethnogynecology, the language women used to describe gynecological complaints, their explanatory models of these problems, their concerns about them, and self-care practices. Over one hundred women (ages 20 to 55) from four villages were interviewed. An additional month of ethnographic research was conducted to collect detailed case histories of fifty women self-reporting chronic or recurrent gynecological complaints.

Interviewing and documentation in ten village grocery shops and twenty pharmacies provided additional data on medication availability, pharmaceutical purchasing patterns for gynecological complaints, and medications marketing. A month of health service research was carried out in three district hospitals, and in three referral clinics/hospitals (the provincial hospital, an MCH hospital, and a VD clinic) in the city of Khon Kaen. Patient flow analysis of women reporting gynecological complaints was conducted, accompanied by 25 exit interviews which probed women's health concerns, expectations from the clinic visit, and perceptions of quality of care. Additional interviews were conducted with health providers at health posts (*sathani anamai*), private practitioners, and village health volunteers.

Ethnogynecology and Explanatory Models of Illness

Ethnographic research revealed that women's discussions of gynecological complaints focused on an area of the body referred to as the *mot luk*. Although the word *mot luk* literally translates as "uterus," ethnogynecological models of the *mot luk* and its associated health problems did not necessarily correspond to biomedical models of anatomy. Women often used the term *mot luk* to refer to the uterus itself, and employed a second term–*pik mot luk*–to refer to its "wings," that is, the parts roughly equivalent to the fallopian tubes and ovaries. When asked to draw diagrams of the *mot luk*, women sometimes drew the *pik mot luk* and *mot luk* separately, with no connection between them. Other women conceived of the uterus as consisting of only the two "wings," with no central portion. Some women explained that there are two *mot luk*, and that male babies develop in the right *mot luk* and female babies in the left. Other women drew diagrams in which the fetus was pictured in the abdomen outside the *mot luk* altogether. Some diagrams depicted the *mot luk* as connected to other bodily channels such as the spine and the stomach.

As locally conceived, *mot luk* problems encompass a wide array of symptoms broadly associated with the reproductive tract, abdominal and pelvic regions, and sometimes the urinary tract. *Mot luk* problems described by local women included symptoms of reproductive tract infections as well as pelvic, lower abdominal and back pains associated with childbearing, menstruation, manual labor, and other symptoms linked to the "uterus" through cultural reasoning. Women frequently referred to symptoms ranging from abdominal and lower back pain to vaginal discharge, itching, odor, and rash using the phrase *pen mot luk* (literally: "it's the uterus"). Local illness terms associated with the uterus included *jep mot luk* ("pain in the uterus"), which is used to refer to abdominal pain of various work-related and reproductive etiologies; *mot luk ak sep* (inflammation/infection of the uterus), an ambiguous term for *mot luk* problems that is sometimes described as simply a more "medical" term for *jep mot luk*; and *mot luk bo di (mot luk mai di)*[2] (bad uterus), which refers to chronic uterine abnormalities with multiple possible causes.

Mot luk problems were believed to have a wide range of causes and a variety of events were considered to make women vulnerable to them. These often included factors that Western medicine would not consider to be related to reproductive physiology. Many women associated their symptoms with hard work, including especially carrying heavy objects, working in rice and sugar cane fields, and weaving. This applies especially to pain (e.g., *jep mot luk*), but hard work was also associated with other symptoms; for example, one woman said that hard work like digging caused her uterus to tear, resulting in *mot luk ak sep* and vaginal discharge. Many women with recurrent symptoms saw their problems as ultimately resulting from some event earlier in life that either caused their ongoing symptoms or made them vulnerable to problems that emerged at a later point in time. Consequential past events included injury or over-work in youth, a complication during a past pregnancy or abortion, pushing too hard during childbirth, and sterilization. More than a quarter of the women interviewed who suffered from chronic or recurrent *mot luk* problems felt that their symptoms were the result of an inadequate period of *yu fai*, the traditional postpartum practice of "staying by the fire" for 10 to 15 days following childbirth, which is said to reposition and dry out the *mot luk* (see also Whittaker 2000).

Various forms of impurities were also considered to be sources of *mot luk* problems. For example, women referred to menstrual blood as *leuat sia* or *leuat bo di* (bad blood), and contrasted the dark color of menstrual blood with "normal" blood which is light red in color. Menstruation was viewed as a monthly cleansing of impurities from the woman's body; if women did not menstruate regularly, or if their menstrual flow was in any way blocked, impurities might remain in the body and result in *mot luk* problems.[3] Women also described symptoms as resulting from *seua la (cheua ra)*, a term that literally translates as "fungus" but is also more broadly associated with dirtiness or germs.

Sources of *seua la* that could cause *mot luk* problems included dirt entering the vagina from sitting on the ground, sweating, not washing the vagina while working all day, wading in dirty water to fish or collect plants, and having sexual intercourse with a husband who engages in extramarital sex. A few women also mentioned a specialized type of *seua la* associated with a particular illness, for example, a germ that eats up the *mot luk*, making an ulcer that can then become cancer. Some women identified two kinds of *seua la*: a contagious discharge-causing *seua la* associated with wetness, and a non-contagious rash-causing *seua la* associated with itching. Informants spoke of women as being particularly susceptible to *seua la* because the vagina is "open" to *seua la* from the exterior world, in contrast to men's genitals which are more "closed."

A number of women with recurrent or chronic symptoms saw their illness as latent. They felt that they experienced recurrent symptoms because the disease or germs remained in their bodies and only manifested themselves at certain times, or because a "wound" (*phe [phle]*) in the uterus persisted without ever entirely healing. *Lok lop nai (rok lop nai)* refers to such illness that "hides" in the body and emerges at times of vulnerability. Hard work, as well as menstruation and fatigue, were the most commonly cited triggers of symptom re-emergence. Some women interpreted vaginal discharge experienced before menses as a latent illness emerging. Others spoke of *seua la* accumulating in the body as a result of poor hygiene or sexual transmission; at times of vulnerability, the *seua la* would emerge as disease.

Many women feared that untreated or chronic symptoms would become a more severe illness. Some women who experienced recurrent symptoms mentioned specific problems that their symptoms might turn into, such as a prolapsed uterus, a tumor, kidney stones, dysuria, or AIDS, while others expressed a non-specific concern that their illness could become "something worse." However, women's greatest concern by far was that their symptoms would "become" cervical cancer (*maleng pak mot luk*, or simply *maleng*).[4] Of fifty women with recurrent symptoms interviewed, 49 believed that the gynecological and abdominal symptoms they experienced could become cancer. Even those who reported that their symptoms were minor thought that they could turn into cancer, and ultimately lead to death (see also Boonmongkon et al. 1999). This perception was reiterated in interviews with health providers. Fears of cervical cancer were a prominent and unexpected theme that emerged recurrently throughout our research. In order to understand the persistent perception that *mot luk* problems can lead to cancer and death, we must turn to the various ways in which the local and the global interact to create new meanings for women.

ILLNESS MANAGEMENT:
INTERFACE BETWEEN THE LOCAL AND THE GLOBAL

Self-Medication

Isan women seek relief from their *mot luk* problems through both self-medication and use of health services. Eighty percent of all women surveyed (n = 1028) reported self-medicating the last time they experienced a *mot luk* problem. Three-quarters of these women purchased their medicines at village grocery shops, and almost two-thirds of them bought antibiotics–most typically, one of two popular brands of tetracycline (Gano® and Hero®).[5] These brands of tetracycline are widely believed to be "good for *mot luk* problems" in general, and also capable of improving the condition of a "bad uterus" (*mot luk bo di [mot luk mai di]*). Some women spoke of these drugs as a cure for common *mot luk* problems, others as a means of preventing *mot luk* problems from becoming worse, others as a prophylactic against the recurrence of problems they had experienced in the past, and still others as a pain killer for *mot luk* problems. Several women compared the ability of antibiotics to dry up excessive vaginal discharge with their ability to dry external wounds.

The use of tetracycline as a cure-all for *mot luk* problems is not merely the result of a global product being appropriated for use by a local population. The pharmaceutical industry has capitalized on local perceptions and used deceptive marketing encouraging the association between tetracycline and *mot luk* problems. Poster and radio advertising employ images that encourage the perception that these drugs are cures for reproductive symptoms (see Boonmongkon et al. 1998; Whittaker 1996). For example, one advertising poster for Gano includes the following elements, with no accompanying explanation: "Gano" written in large letters, male and female icons (possibly implying STD treatment), and a picture of a uterus. Thus, the way in which tetracycline is used for *mot luk* problems represents a bidirectional interface between local conceptions and global products mediated through marketing practices.

Hybrid Ideas Relating to Women's Interactions with the Health Sector

When self-medication fails to decrease the severity of a *mot luk* problem or when a problem is recurrent, women often visit a government clinic. Government health posts (*sathani anamai*) staffed by nurses and/or midwives are found in most larger villages and within clusters of smaller adjoining villages. District hospitals are found in most towns. Nursing staff at local health posts and district hospitals see approximately three-quarters of all women in their service areas at least once per year. In the past year, 47 percent of women we surveyed (n = 1028) had visited a government health facility for some service related to obstetrics and gynecology (family planning, pre- or postnatal care, Pap smears, or *mot luk* problems). Eighty percent of women in the community survey who consulted some practitioner for a gynecological complaint they deemed serious visited a government health facility and 34 percent a private practitioner–most after consulting a government practitioner first.

Women's expectations of government health services were strongly influenced by both longstanding ideas about the body and illness, and emerging health concerns triggered by global health initiatives and national health programs. These women's understandings of their illness experiences may best be characterized as hybrid. Hybrid ideas about health and illness often emerge when adequate explanations for health provider actions or inaction are not forthcoming, and patients attempt to make sense of their health problems by extending familiar conceptual frameworks to their new circumstances. Their existing conceptions then become transformed in the process of incorporating new information that emerges through interactions with the health sector. In this study, we found that hybrid ideas resulted from the intersection of existing conceptualizations of health, emerging concerns about vulnerability and risk associated with health education, and practitioner responses to health care needs negotiated in local health arenas. Below, we describe Isan women's response to a Pap smear campaign introduced in Khon Kaen Province. The case is instructive because it illustrates what can happen when a well-meaning public health program is introduced without attention to popular health culture.

Fears of Cervical Cancer and Health Education

Almost all informants suffering recurrent symptoms (n = 50) believed that their *mot luk* problems could eventually lead to cervical cancer (*maleng pak mot luk*), or simply cancer (*maleng*). The connection that women drew between a wide range of abdominal and reproductive tract symptoms and cervical cancer can be explained by looking at their ethnomedical model of what is happening inside their bodies. From a biomedical perspective, women's complaints of *mot luk* problems may include fungal, viral or bacterial infections that may be sexually transmitted as well as endogenous or iatrogenic in origin (Sobel 1989; Tsui et al. 1997), and muscle strain associated with hard manual labor. Each problem is different and requires specific treatment. Women in this study, however, saw things differently. They placed a wide range of *mot luk* problems on the same illness continuum as cervical cancer (see also Whittaker 2000). The visual images of *mot luk* problems that most women described included the presence of a large ulcer, fungus, or collection of pus inside the uterus. They had a macroscopic rather than microscopic image of the problem; that is, they imagined a large uterine anomaly that would be visible to the naked eye upon inspection during an internal exam. Cervical cancer was imagined as an extreme, life-threatening stage in the development of this uterine anomaly–the final common outcome of all untreated *mot luk* problems.

While there were many different, and often ambiguous, ideas about how *mot luk* symptoms can progress through stages and eventually become cervical cancer, the image of an ulcer, fungus/germ, pus, or "infection" inside the uterus was a common theme. The specific, imagined pathways leading from women's own symptoms to cancer varied from woman to woman, but included certain common ideas. The initial symptoms were often described as *jep mot luk* (pain in the uterus), *jep thong noi* (lower abdominal pain), *mot luk ak sep* (inflammation/infection of the uterus), *mot luk bo di* (bad uterus), or *mat khaw* (vaginal discharge); in some cases, these problems were believed to lead directly to cancer, whereas in others they were imagined to cause a secondary set of symptoms, including discharge, fungus, itching, an ulcer or tumor, or infection, which then becomes cancer. For example, women made statements such as: "*Mot luk bo di* causes discharge, and if you have a lot of discharge, you will eventually get cancer"; "If you work hard you will get *mot luk ak sep*, and if you have *mot luk ak sep* for a long time, it will cause a tumor which will become cancer"; and "If a man has extramarital sex, he can give his wife *seua la* (fungus/germs), which will then make an ulcer inside the uterus that becomes cancer."[6] Regardless of the particular series of intermediate stages, all informants recognized cervical cancer as the final common outcome.

The rate of cervical cancer in Thailand is estimated to be 28 cases per 100,000 women. Yet interviews revealed an expectation among informants that 9 to 16% of women over age 25 in their communities would develop cancer, equivalent to 9 to 16 *thousand* cases per 100,000 women. The ethnophysiological models of the relationship between *mot luk* problems and cervical cancer described above partially account for this exaggerated perception of risk. Ideas presented in health education materials distributed as part of a cervical cancer screening campaign in the area have been appropriated by women and incorporated into these pre-existing, ethnogynecological perceptions, and have thus come to inadvertently reinforce such local models. One educational poster showing an enlarged photograph of advanced cervical cancer provided women with a macro-image of a microscopic anomaly; with no indication as to the scale of the photograph, the picture bears a striking resemblance to a large ulcer, fungus, or accumulation of pus. This image thus served to reinforce the existing visual model of cervical cancer and perpetuated the link between cancer and the imagined manifestations of *mot luk* problems (Boonmongkon et al. 1998, 2001).

In the context of concerns that a wide range of *mot luk* problems may potentially transform into fatal cervical cancer, the intensive cervical cancer awareness and screening campaign conducted in this region has inadvertently heightened these fears. The impact of health education activities was evident from in-depth interviews conducted with women who suffered from recurrent symptoms. One woman stated that, from the health education messages dispersed over the village loudspeaker, she learned how common cervical cancer is among women her age, and it made her so afraid of cancer that she suffers from insomnia. Several women reported going to the local health post to request sleeping pills because worrying about cancer kept them awake at night. One woman explicitly stated that her symptoms were not serious enough to prevent her from working as usual, but that she was still worried about them turning into cervical cancer *because they conducted a health education campaign in her village*. Another woman commented that "years ago people did not know about cervical cancer. Women had [vaginal] discharge and thought they had syphilis or gonorrhea. Now we think, cancer."

Psychological suffering from such worry and fear manifests itself as anxiety, insomnia, worry about chronic illness or death in the future, and concern over who will take care of children when chronic illness prevents the woman from fulfilling this role. Yet the great majority of these women most likely suffer from non-life threatening conditions such as recurrent bacterial or fungal infections that might be easily managed, if not cured.

Fears of Cancer and Practitioner Diagnosis of Mot luk Ak sep

Mot luk ak sep (infection/inflammation of the uterus) is a widely used but rather indiscriminate local term employed by women to speak about a persistent *mot luk* problem. Despite its lack of specificity, more than a quarter of the women interviewed reported that a doctor or health worker had told them they had *mot luk ak sep* (and sometimes *mot luk bo di*, a "bad uterus"). For the most part, no additional explanation accompanied this diagnosis. Use of the term provided practitioners with a flexible label for a woman's health problem when symptoms were not clear or when treatment had been ineffective. Some practitioners also noted that this diagnosis allowed them to describe a complex condition using a term that the patient would understand. When health care providers used the term *mot luk ak sep* without offering a patient any indication as to what was abnormal about her uterus, many patients interpreted this to mean that they had a problem that was likely to escalate. Given recent health promotion activities associated with cervical cancer, many women feared that the problems in their uteri might be progressing to cervical cancer. Thus, in appropriating the term *mot luk ak sep* and using it as a "specifically ambiguous" diagnosis (Nichter 1989, 1997), health care providers left women with unresolved doubts about their health problems, as well as a heightened feeling of fear associated with cervical cancer.

Concerns About Mot luk Problems and Use of Pap Smear Services

Increasing awareness of cervical cancer in Khon Kaen Province has led to both higher cervical cancer screening rates and heightened fears. Our community survey (n = 1028) indicated that 35% of women had received a Pap smear within the past two years. Yet while women were indeed responding to the campaign by engaging cervical cancer screening services, their ideas about the purpose of a Pap smear, and their associated reasons for attending Pap smear clinics, did not correspond to the global, medical conception of a Pap smear as a preventive, screening procedure for healthy women. Rather, their use of Pap smear clinics was frequently linked to *mot luk* problems and associated concerns that existing symptoms could turn into cervical cancer.

District hospitals offer weekly Pap smear clinics. We observed that when women complaining of gynecological symptoms visited a district hospital and requested an "internal exam," they were often asked by the nurse at the patient triage counter to go to the hospital's Pap smear clinic or come back on a Pap smear clinic day. Medical staff thus treated them as if they were coming in for cervical cancer screening, and in many cases women were sent home without questions being asked about their problems and without treatment being administered, unless symptoms were very severe. Pap smears were generally conducted by nursing staff in the health promotion section of the hospital, but reproductive tract infections were not treated by nursing staff conducting these exams. Furthermore, patients were poorly informed about the purpose of a Pap smear. They understood a Pap smear as a *diagnostic* procedure for all *mot luk* problems (the worst of which is cancer), not a *screening* procedure for precursors of cervical cancer. Since many women thought of cervical cancer as a large ulcer, fungus, or accumulation of pus that would be visible to the naked eye upon inspection, they expected to be immediately diagnosed when examined. However, instead of being informed by nursing staff about what they had seen, they were told to wait for laboratory results that often took up to three months to process. Thus, women's expectations for diagnosis and treatment were not met, and they went away worried, unsatisfied, and untreated.

Survey data revealed that of the 356 women who had received a Pap smear within the past two years, 151 (42%) sought out the service *because they were experiencing abnormal symptoms.* The majority of other women had been recruited directly by health workers. Consistent with the finding that women who attended Pap smear clinics did so because they had abnormal symptoms, we found that half of the women in our survey (n = 1028) who did not go for cervical cancer screening gave "no abnormal symptoms" as a primary reason for not going.[7] Women's use of Pap smear clinics thus reflects a hybrid understanding of the purpose of Pap smear services, a perception which draws from both the global discourse of cervical cancer screening, and the local discourse of *mot luk* problems and their relationship to cancer. The consequences of this hybrid understanding are both a potential under-use of cervical cancer screening by healthy women, and ineffective treatment as well as patient dissatisfaction where women with *mot luk* problems expect their symptoms to be diagnosed and treated upon presentation at a Pap smear clinic.

STAGE TWO:
TRANSLATING RESEARCH INTO PRACTICE

In stage two of the project, five sub-district health posts, three district hospitals and one village having an active health volunteer group were selected as sites for piloting an integrated set of women's health interventions. Interventions were designed to be gender and culturally sensitive, taking into account what had been learned during stage one research. In keeping with formative research principles, all intervention activities were carefully monitored by research staff to facilitate midcourse correction. The following is a brief description of some of the interventions implemented between 1998-2001 as well as lessons learned.

Creation of Culturally-Appropriate IEC Materials

A majority of Isan women under 45 are either literate or have a literate neighbor they can turn to as a confidant. Information, education, and communication (IEC) pamphlets and posters were developed to address women's health concerns identified during stage one research. A key feature of these materials was a question and answer format anticipating questions women were likely to have based on points of confusion documented during stage one. To date, guides to understanding vaginal discharge, *mot luk* problems and abdominal pain, prolapsed uterus, cervical cancer, and urinary tract problems have been pre-tested and made available to rural women at government health clinics and rural health posts. The pamphlets are in high demand by women, and nurses find them to be a useful resource. Unlike other health materials distributed to the community and soon discarded, women have been found to keep and refer to project materials when problems arise. Nurses have been observed to use the written materials as well as plastic models of female anatomy we supplied when discussing health problems with patients. There is also evidence that reading pamphlets has influenced women's health communication with nurses. According to nurses at local health posts, women who have read IEC materials tend to ask more questions and offer more detailed histories. Exposure to the question and answer format featured in the IEC pamphlets fosters patient-nurse communication.

Community Outreach

In a pilot village, sixteen reproductive health volunteers (8 women and 8 men) have been trained to deliver health messages about reproductive and sexual health to their neighbors and to promote village-wide dialogue about gender and sexual health issues. The volunteers underwent several days of intensive training incorporating local notions of ethnophysiology, illness causality and self-care practices. Volunteers were provided with medical knowledge about reproductive health and encouraged to act as cultural brokers, helping neighbors to better understand their health problems. It has been the task of project staff to both encourage creative thought and monitor emergent ideas, so that misconceptions may be corrected in a culturally sensitive manner. For example, during one session, a female volunteer suggested that if a woman underwent a tubectomy she did not have to worry about AIDS because the virus could not move up her body beyond her blocked tubes. Correcting such misconceptions at the level of health volunteers is essential, since they serve as a gateway for health information distribution within the village.

Volunteer training has been practical and based on real life situations documented during formative research. The most effective forms of volunteer training have involved interactive problem solving exercises using storytelling, drama, and role-play. For example, sensitive gender relations issues have been approached from the perspective that social relations vary across different couples. Volunteers are asked to come up with several different ways of resolving a problem and then discuss what type of solution might be best for different people, an exercise inspired by self-efficacy theory (Bandura 1998). Many of the scenarios used in problem solving exercises were based upon the research conducted during stage one of the project. Volunteers have also been trained to go over IEC materials with their neighbors. They report that these materials boost their credibility as purveyors of knowledge. Visual props such as inexpensive aprons depicting body organs, an idea borrowed from a reproductive health project in Malaysia, have been helpful and fun for villagers. Volunteers wear an organ map apron when talking about anatomy, physiology and pathology. Teams of one male and one female reproductive health volunteer visit households in the evening and invite discussion about sexual and reproductive health topics. Sometimes husbands and wives are spoken to separately and at other times together.

Village-wide events have also raised the visibility of volunteer activities. For example, a health fair was held where villagers had the opportunity to talk to visiting health care providers about their problems. Health providers acknowledged health volunteers when answering questions. The most successful event during the health fair was a quiz show on reproductive health. This format drew on the popularity of television quiz shows in Isan. Questions were asked about issues in the IEC materials and key messages volunteers had been promoting. Participants in the game won prizes, and since the same question appeared several times during the quiz, the audience was very attentive.

During village level meetings attended and videotaped by the research team, volunteers have been far more open to discussing sexual health than the team had originally anticipated. In addition to questions about illness and new medications available at the local health posts (such as vaginal tablets), villagers have discussed such sensitive issues as the side effects of sex potions which tighten a woman's vagina for the purpose of pleasing her husband, women's response to men who swell the head size of their penis by inserting smooth pieces of glass, and the waning of sexual desire during aging. The research team has found that once rapport with the community has been established, sexual health is not a taboo subject. The project has given people the space to openly discuss topics normally considered private.

Health Post and Clinic-Based Interventions

Nursing staff from all rural health posts and district hospitals in the project area have been provided training to upgrade both their technical and cultural communication skills. Our research suggested that nurses previously offered women irrational treatment for *mot luk* problems (see Boonmongkon et al. 1998). This was due to both a lack of knowledge and a lack of appropriate medicines. In stage two, nurses were introduced to a syndromic approach to diagnosis and treatment of common reproductive tract infections. Syndromic treatment algorithms used in the training were modified from WHO materials so as to better match the Thai epidemiological profile.[8] The focus of Thai nurse undergraduate training is on the recognition of serious upper reproductive tract infections (such a syphilis and gonorrhea). During the project, more emphasis was placed on the treatment of more common lower reproductive tract infections such as fungal infections and bacterial vaginosis. Nurses were taught how and when to use anti-fungal vaginal tablets and metronidazole, two drugs previously not supplied to rural health posts and only available at district hospitals.[9] Nurses were further taught how best to manage pelvic and muscle pain associated with hard manual labor. Considerable attention was placed on how to conduct a culturally sensitive patient history and physical exam.

During cultural training, nurses were introduced to the concept of reproductive health and sensitized to think beyond disease to women's experience of illness and how it affects their everyday lives. Data collected during our formative research were reviewed during the first day of training to ground nurses in popular health culture. Nurses were then asked to participate in a series of role-playing exercises in which they explored ways of identifying and talking to women about their doubts and concerns. Attention was paid to the language of illness and patients' interpretation of practitioners' use of the terms *mot luk ak sep* and *mot luk bo di* which lead to miscommunication. Women's fear of cancer was discussed at length, as were local understandings of Pap smears and patient expectations from nurses following an internal exam.

According to the findings of an ongoing observational study, there has been a notable improvement in the quality of care offered to Isan women by nurses participating in the project. Most health posts now have weekly reproductive health clinic days when Pap smears are conducted and all health posts in the project area have changed their physical layout to ensure patient privacy during internal examinations. Nurses treat women with *mot luk* problems more conscientiously and communication with patients has improved significantly. In-depth case records are kept for women with chronic or recurrent complaints and a better referral system has been set in motion. Health post nurses who refer patients to the district hospital are now far more likely to receive feedback about a patient's diagnosis and treatment, enabling them to follow-up and manage care plans. Time from receiving a Pap smear exam to securing the results of the exam has also decreased significantly. Prior to the project it was not uncommon for women to receive the results of their tests two to three months after the exam. This time period has been shortened to less than a month and at some health posts provisions have been made so that women may pay a modest fee to receive prompt results from a private lab in Khon Kaen city.

THE CHALLENGES AHEAD

The international health literature is replete with successful pilot projects that could not be sustained or go to scale. If the present women's health project is to be a catalyst for change, it will need to build a network of interested reproductive health care providers who are capable of serving as role models, enabling the reproductive health program to gradually expand to scale. This requires sustaining the interest of a critical mass of nurses through periodic meetings, training exercises, and mentorship activities. Exemplary health posts are presently being considered as possible training sites for both the next generation of nurses (nursing students at Khon Kaen Nursing school undergoing their practica) as well as nurses presently stationed at health posts yet to be covered by the project. We originally envisioned that experienced health post nurses might play a leadership role in technical and cultural training activities for new groups of nurses. However, ongoing formative research has suggested that nurses sharing the same professional status are uncomfortable receiving training from each other, even if the latter have received additional training. While exemplary nurses may serve as mentors for those being trained, training facilitators will need to be of higher status in the health care hierarchy.

In Thailand, health care reform at the district level is likely to be uneven despite changes in national health policy because district medical officers retain a degree of power and autonomy. An ongoing challenge faced by project staff has been to learn how to facilitate change in different management environments. For example, while a participatory bottom-up approach to the planning of a reproductive health clinic was feasible in one district hospital in the project area because the doctor in charge maintained good relations with community leaders, in the next district there was virtually no contact between the head doctor and community leaders. All decisions about reproductive health activities were thus made in a top-down manner with the project team serving as a liaison to the community. Health care reform activities need to be undertaken in different environments, with the hope that successful models of health care delivery will inspire future health care planning.

DISCUSSION

The case study presented here illustrates a proactive means by which to work toward women's health care reform. An important part of the action research process described has been an ethnographic investigation of reproductive health as it is locally understood, and a gender sensitive appraisal of the social relations of health care delivery. These assessments are just as important to health care reform as the analysis of epidemiological data on disease prevalence and health systems data on cost effectiveness. We wish to further emphasize that formative research into popular health culture and patient-provider interactions should not be seen as a one-time research effort prior to the development of culturally and gender sensitive health services. Popular health culture is dynamic and interactions between local and global sources of knowledge and influence are bound to have a wide range of unanticipated and ongoing effects.

In this paper we have provided a case which illustrates why it is important to monitor popular health culture and take hybrid knowledge seriously. Isan women's heightened concern about cervical cancer in Khon Kaen Province is an emergent phenomenon. It is linked to the way in which the local population has interpreted health communication about Pap smears within the context of pre-existing ideas about ethnogynecology and illness etiology. This case of iatrogenic fear of cervical cancer is instructive for two reasons. Firstly, it documents how a public health campaign focusing on only one women's health problem may backfire, drawing attention to the need for a more comprehensive women's health package. Secondly, it illustrates why health social scientists are needed to monitor public health interventions over time.

Raising community awareness about the risk of cervical cancer has been successful in motivating women to accept Pap smears in Khon Kaen Province, but at what cost? Fear has clearly placed women at a higher risk for suffering. One might argue that letting women live with the dread of cancer when they are only suffering from fungal infections or occupational health problems is against the medical dictum to "do no harm." We would argue that public health, like medicine, needs to be held accountable for what transpires when health messages are introduced into the community. Likewise, the pharmaceutical industry needs to be held accountable for how medicines are being used by a population as a result of marketing and distribution practices. The popularity of tetracycline in self-medication for gynecological problems in Khon Kaen Province is as much a result of marketing as cultural perceptions of medicines. Given a steady stream of global health information and products from both the private and public sectors, ongoing formative research, and especially ethnography, is needed to inform health care reform.

NOTES

1. For a comprehensive description of research methods and our formative research model, see Boonmongkon et al. 1998.

2. In this paper, we transcribe Isan terms into the Roman alphabet according to local pronunciation; that is, our spelling corresponds to the ways in which people speaking the Isan (Lao) dialect pronounce words rather than to central Thai spelling conventions. However, since this Lao-speaking population lives within the Thai nation-state, their speech is influenced by central Thai, and they therefore engage in frequent code-

switching, interspersing Thai terms and pronunciations with Isan patterns. The use of central Thai interviewers in this research likely influenced respondents to engage in such code-switching as well. We therefore include, in parentheses following Isan terms, any alternate terms and pronunciations from the central Thai dialect that were commonly used by respondents. This transcription system does not indicate vowel length or tones.

3. Further evidence of this belief comes from a study in Northern Thailand, where it has been found that women who are HIV positive are believed to develop AIDS symptoms less quickly and live longer than men because menstruation has the effect of purifying women's blood every month (Chongsathitmun et al. 2000:225).

4. Similarly, Bang et al. (1989) report that, in India, women believed that vaginal discharge could progress from mild to severe forms, causing a gradual deterioration in health leading to weakness and eventual death. Visual, gastric, urinary, and sexual problems, as well as sterility and cancer were some specific, potential consequences associated with discharge.

5. Most women self-medicated by using one to three pills of tetracycline, an inadequate dose. Even when taken in the correct dosage, this medicine is inappropriate for muscle pain and fungal infections. Fungal infections are in fact exacerbated by the use of antibiotics.

6. Similar variability in the perceived causes of cervical cancer has been found among Latina immigrants in the United States, one of the few populations for which such data exist (see Chavez et al. 1995; Hubbell et al. 1996).

7. An association between Pap smears and abnormal symptoms is consistent with the findings of Wood et al. (1997) in a study of women of color in South Africa. As in the current study, these authors found that most women who received Pap smears initially went to a health facility with gynecological symptoms. However, in contrast to the findings of our study, reproductive tract infections were often identified, diagnosed and treated during internal exams in conjunction with Pap smears. Treatment further reinforced women's perception that Pap smears were a diagnostic tool for identifying gynecological disease. The authors found that opportunistic screening of women who sought family planning services further resulted in an association between cervical cancer screening and contraception.

8. Case management guidelines for *mot luk* and reproductive tract problems were prepared and pre-tested by the Department of Communicable Diseases Control, MOPH of Thailand. The flowcharts focus on diagnosis and treatment of vaginal discharge, discharge from the urethra, lower abdominal pain, ulcers of the reproductive organs, and prolapsed uterus.

9. District hospitals supplied gynecon, clotrimazole and metronidazole tablets as well as clotrimazole cream from their stocks, enabling nurses at health posts to treat trichomonas, candidiasis, and bacterial vaginitis.

REFERENCES

Bandura, A. (1998). Health promotion from the perspective of social cognitive theory. *Psychology and Health* 13, 623-649.

Bang, R.A., Bang, A.T., Baitule, M., Choudhary, Y., Sarmukaddam, S., and O. Tale (1989). High prevalence of gynaecological diseases in rural Indian women. *Lancet* (January 14), 85-88.

Boonmongkon, P., Nichter, M., and J. Pylypa (2001). *Mot luk* problems in Northeast Thailand: why women's own health concerns matter as much as disease rates. *Social Science and Medicine* 53, 1095-1112.

Boonmongkon, P., Nichter, M., Pylypa, J., and K. Chantapasa (1998). *Understanding Women's Experience of Gynecological Problems: An Ethnographic Case Study from Northeast Thailand.* Nakornpathom: Center for Health Policy Studies, Mahidol University.

Boonmongkon, P., Pylypa, J., and M. Nichter (1999). Emerging fears of cervical cancer in Northeast Thailand. *Anthropology and Medicine* 16(4), 359-380.

Chavez, L.R., Hubbell, F.A., McMullin, J.M., Martinez, R.G., and S.I. Mishra (1995). Structure and meaning in models of breast and cervical cancer risk factors: a comparison of perceptions among Latinas, Anglo women, and physicians. *Medical Anthropology Quarterly* 9(1), 40-74.

Chongsathitmun, J., Atthamet, R., and P. Chukping (2000). Gender, sexuality, reproductive health in Northern Thailand: literature review. *Journal of Social Sciences* 12(1), 225.

DeJong, J. (2000). The role of the Cairo International Conference on Population and Development. *Social Science and Medicine* 51, 941-953.

Ginsburg, F.D. and R. Rapp (eds.) (1995). *Conceiving the New World Order: The Global Politics of Reproduction.* Berkeley: University of California Press.

Hardee, K., Agarwal, K., Luke, N., Wilson, E., Pendzich, M., Farrell, M., and H. Cross (1999). Reproductive Health Policies and Programs in Eight Countries: Progress Since Cairo. *International Family Planning Perspectives* 25, S2-S9.

Hempel, M. (1996). Reproductive health and rights: origins and challenges to the ICPD agenda. *Health Transition Review* 6, 73-85.

Hubbell, F.A., Chavez, L.R., Mishra, S.I., and R.B. Valdez (1996). Beliefs about sexual behavior and other predictors of Papanicolaou smear screening among Latinas and Anglo women. *Archives of Internal Medicine* 156, 2353-2358.

Nichter, M. (1989). The language of disease. In Nichter, M., *Anthropology and International Health* (First Edition). Dordrecht: Kluwer Press, pp. 83-123.

Nichter, M. (1997). Illness semantics and international health: the weak lungs/TB complex in the Philippines. In Inhorn, M., Brown, P. (eds.), *Anthropology and Infectious Disease.* Amsterdam: Gordon and Breach Publishers, pp. 267-298.

Sadana, R. (2000). Measuring reproductive health: review of community based approaches to assessing morbidity. *Bulletin of the World Health Organization* 78(5), 640-654.

Sobel, J.D. (1989). Bacterial vaginosis–an ecologic mystery. *Annals of Internal Medicine* 111(7), 551-552.

Tsui, A.O., Wasserheit, J.N., and J.G. Haaga (eds.) (1997). *Reproductive Health in Developing Countries: Expanding Dimensions, Building Solutions.* Washington, DC, National Academy Press.

Whittaker, A. (1996). White blood and falling wombs: ethnogynecology in Northeast Thailand. In Rice, P.L., Manderson, L. (eds.), *Maternity and Reproductive Health in Asian Societies.* Amsterdam: Harwood Academic Publishers, pp. 207-225.

Whittaker, A. (2000). *Intimate Knowledge: Women and Their Health in North-East Thailand.* Sydney: Allen and Unwin.

WHO (World Health Organization) (1999). Interpreting Reproductive Health. (WHO\CHS\RHR\99.7). Geneva: WHO.

Wood, K., Jewkes, R., and N. Abrahams (1997). Cleaning the womb: constructions of cervical screening and womb cancer among rural Black women in South Africa. *Social Science and Medicine* 45(2), 283-294.

Menstrual Madness:
Women's Health and Well-Being
in Urban Burma

Monique Skidmore, MA, PhD

SUMMARY. Women's health in peri-urban Burma is conceived of in terms of blood, strength, and the relationship between the body, the body politic, and the local environment. The regulation and volume of blood at menstruation and childbirth are the fundamental indicators of health and well-being. Well-being is contingent on harmony in and between the body and the universe. Blood flow is a key symbol through which women's beliefs and practices concerning their health and well-being can be understood at the levels of pathophysiology, interpersonal relations, the local environment, and the wider political and moral economies of urban Burma. *[Article copies available for a fee from The Haworth Document Delivery Service: 1-800-HAWORTH. E-mail address: <getinfo@ haworthpressinc.com> Website: <http://www.HaworthPress.com> © 2002 by The Haworth Press, Inc. All rights reserved.]*

KEYWORDS. Burma, Myanmar, women, health, menstruation, abortion, body, body politic

Monique Skidmore is Lecturer, School of Anthropology, Geography and Environmental Studies, The University of Melbourne, Victoria, 3010, Australia (E-mail: mskid@unimelb.edu.au).

Funding for the fieldwork on which this paper is based was provided by the Wenner-Gren Fund for Anthropological Research (Grant No. 6049), The Social Sciences Council of McGill University, and a University of Melbourne Career Research Establishment Grant.

[Haworth co-indexing entry note]: "Menstrual Madness: Women's Health and Well-Being in Urban Burma." Skidmore, Monique. Co-published simultaneously in *Women & Health* (The Haworth Medical Press, an imprint of The Haworth Press, Inc.) Vol. 35, No. 4, 2002, pp. 81-99; and: *Women's Health in Mainland Southeast Asia* (ed: Andrea Whittaker) The Haworth Medical Press, an imprint of The Haworth Press, Inc., 2002, pp. 81-99. Single or multiple copies of this article are available for a fee from The Haworth Document Delivery Service [1-800-HAWORTH, 9:00 a.m. - 5:00 p.m. (EST). E-mail address: getinfo@ haworthpressinc.com].

INTRODUCTION

Sweat runs from my hair and spills down my neck onto the rough-hewn concrete floor. I look to the banana and breadfruit trees, hoping for evidence of a slight breeze. It is only eight a.m. in the morning. The mango trees are heavy with fruit not yet ripe. I squint at the painfully bright sky, waiting for a hint of cloud, a sign that the mango showers have arrived. It is early May, the hottest part of the dry season. Within a few days the mango showers will begin in the afternoons. The mangoes themselves will become yellow and fragrant and a collective sigh of relief will be breathed with the knowledge that the hot season will soon be replaced with the wet season.

It is 1997 and I am sitting in a schoolhouse with a group of women who are teaching me the links between daily events, illnesses, and socioeconomic conditions. Two hundred women were divided into twenty focus groups. Women from each focus group later participated in in-depth qualitative interviews. We have cut-out cardboard circles, each representing a common complaint or illness, and the women are now weaving a causal web between the domains. The women are from peri-urban townships bordering Rangoon,[1] the capital city, and in previous months the same process has been undertaken in Mandalay's peri-urban townships.[2] The four hundred women of reproductive age interviewed at these two fieldwork sites constitute part of a broad range of ethnographic fieldwork conducted in 1994, 1996-7 and 2001.[3]

The most consistent finding arising from the fieldwork data is that the regularity and volume of blood at menstruation and childbirth is the fundamental indicator of health and well-being for women in peri-urban Burma. Being in good health is contingent on harmony in and between the body and the universe, where the latter includes the socioeconomic and political dimensions of everyday life. In the first section of this paper, I demonstrate that blood flow is the key symbol (following Good, 1977) by which Burmese women's beliefs and practices concerning their well-being can be understood. To this end I describe the common categories of "women's illnesses," focusing upon the emmenagogue "thwe-ze."

The next section of the paper examines the way that this generic Burmese pathophysiology is used in the relocated peri-urban townships to experience and express the experience of illness and being unwell. Abortion, childbirth, madness, and "weakness" are the major domains in which I trace understandings of the way that blood flows through the body and how this gives coherence to women's illness, treatment and local etiologies.

In the final section of the paper, I broaden the analysis of women's health as articulated at the levels of pathophysiology, interpersonal relations, and the local peri-urban environment, to include the wider political and moral economies of Burma. All of the women interviewed are adamant that the body, mind, and soul cannot be well if the physical, political, and spiritual domains are not aligned in harmony. The data from this study provide evidence that the moral economy of political dictatorship and the enforced economic impoverishment of the majority of peri-urban Burmans are underlying causes of ill health in general, and of peri-urban "women's diseases" in particular.

BACKGROUND

The causal diagrams drawn by the women trace menstrual antecedents, treatment and the possible outcomes of "women's diseases" in peri-urban Burma. Paul Farmer (1992) has argued that the main risk factor for disease is poverty, a statement certainly borne out by the fieldwork data. High living costs, not having enough money for basic necessities, large families, and frequent hunger caused by having only two inadequate meals per day, are some of the reasons given by the women as precursors of illness. In this section I show how these broad socio-economic conditions are directly related to the current political situation.

Following the failed democracy uprising in August, 1988, the new military council (the State Law and Order Restoration Council) began a major reshaping of Burmese urban centers. The aim of this reorganization was firstly, to isolate those neighborhoods and families thought to be sympathetic to democracy, and secondly, to make room for the growth of a "modern" urban center, much in the way that Baron Haussman remodeled Paris in the 1930s (Buck-Morss, 1989). To achieve these aims the new military council forcibly relocated certain townships and residents to rice paddies on the outskirts of Rangoon and Mandalay. This area has become known as the "New Fields." Some of the wards within these townships incorporate existing small villages. These wards now include farmers who have been dispossessed of their land and who have few skills that allow them to earn a living now that they can no longer farm their land. Urban residents were moved to these areas in army trucks and were often supplied with tin for roofing and sometimes an amount of cash for bamboo walls and flooring.

Originally these townships had no services such as safe water supplies, and only minimal house-building materials. In the last decade the Burmese government has provided township medical offices and a small number of health centers. International aid agencies run programs to improve maternal and child health. In some relocated townships, the government has established "industrial zones" that provide low paying manual labor jobs that have alleviated the chronic unemployment and underemployment of these townships. In other townships, however, there is no industrial zone and unemployment remains extremely high. This had resulted in a very high mobility rate of the population, especially young men, who travel long distances (such as to gem mines) to find employment.

The architecture of the townships differs according to whether they were established around prior villages, which gives a natural center to the township, or on unsettled farmland. Most of the townships did not incorporate villages and their structure most often fans out from a central square. The central square can become either a playing field or a market. It is bordered by the local security office and any other government offices or small shops that have been established, and sometimes teashops. Forced labor was used to create the roads and other infrastructure in the townships.

There is almost no formal employment within the relocated townships. The peri-urban areas ringing Mandalay have, however, many small informal businesses. Livestock can be seen in the streets and compounds, and there is a myriad of individual household productive activities. Such activities include smithing, weaving, basket making, small animal husbandry, rose farming, the recycling of plastic bags, and the recycling of charcoal into small balls.

BURMESE PATHOPHYSIOLOGY

Menstrual regulation and fertility regulation receive little cross-cultural attention except as a form of abortion (Kulczycki et al. 1996; Van de Walle 1997; Singh 1998). Very few studies attempt to place menstrual regulation within local pathophysiological concepts and broader socioeconomic and political frameworks (noticeable exceptions are Sobo 1996; Nations et al. 1997; Whittaker 2000). In this section I situate menstrual and fertility regulation within local understandings of the body and of blood flow. In later sections, I expand this analysis to economic and national issues.

Miyet yawga is glossed, in Burmese, as "women's disease." The expression begins with the word *mi*, or fire, denoting the dangerous nature of women's diseases. Many Burmese women differentiate between a variety of conditions that fall under this rubric. *Miyet sa*, for example, is used to describe many illnesses that are thought to occur with the onset of puberty. Similarly, *miyet pwa* is a term used to describe many illnesses that occur following childbirth. *Miyet yawga* is used specifically to refer to illness within the postpartum period, but has come to be used as the generic term for all of these "women's diseases."[4] *Miyet soh* is used to describe illnesses occurring around the menopause and *miyet youn* describes madness stemming from women's diseases. There is a very common Burmese saying: "*miyet sa, miyet leh, miyet soh.*" The literal translation for *sa* is beginning, for *leh*, is middle, and for *soh*, is end. The saying demonstrates how women's reproductive health is chronologically divided into three periods beginning with puberty. The middle period is filled with pregnancies, and menopause signals the end of the reproductive cycle. The illnesses associated with each of these periods, although often grouped as *miyet yawga*, are understood as separate conditions and have their own etiologies, duration and treatment regimes. There is also a belief that *miyet yawga* can be spread among women in close contact, either through living or working together.

There is another way in which these categories of indigenous disease can be classified. The first, *miyet gan kaiq* concerns illnesses caused by irregularity or insufficient blood flow, and the second, *miyet win kaiq* concerns illnesses caused by excessive blood flow. As I show in following sections, irregular menstruation and amenorrhea are common at all stages of the female reproductive cycle, but especially at menopause. Emmenagogues (known throughout Burma as *thwe-ze*)[5] are often used, in conjunction with diet or contraceptive injections, to restart or strengthen blood flow.

Illnesses caused by too much blood flow are considered to be equally injurious to health; they occur most often after childbirth, miscarriage, and attempted abortions. Diet manipulation is the main method used to staunch bleeding but, increasingly, hemorrhaging women are presenting to local and urban hospitals.

There are several other commonalities with all of these women's illnesses. One is the sequence of treatment regimes now instituted by women seeking help for perceived menstrual irregularities as biomedical health facilities are slowly incorporated into the urban and peri-urban infrastructure. A second is the relatively coherent agreement of several hundred female informants of a Burmese pathophysiology and a rationality that links cause and effect. I introduce this pathophysiology below using Ma Cho Cho's[6] example:

Vignette 1

> Women think that it is very important to bleed. If you don't [bleed], the blood becomes rotten and comes upward and anything can happen. So it needs to come out thoroughly and you need to get rid of the rotten things. You can have a fever, a puffy face, and your skin can become dry, or have dry patches on it or different pigmentations. You become dizzy which means that it's affecting your head. Your stomach will get a solid lump in it.

Ma Cho Cho is a middle-aged woman, portly, with a love of food and an enduring and passionate love for her husband to whom she has been married for more than twenty years. In the vignette above she relates to me her understanding of the more serious problems that can occur if women's diseases are left untreated. Her narrative is revealing for the elements of a distinctly Burmese pathophysiology that are evident in the attribution of symptoms to diseases processes.

Blood is not conceptualized as circulating around the body with the heart acting as a pump. Rather, blood must flow strongly and regularly through the body much as a river must flow through a canyon without becoming blocked by boulders or debris. The lack of blood flow or the cessation of menstruation indicates that blood is not flowing and may be congealing. If treatment is not successful, the blood can solidify inside the stomach and it is conceptualized as forming a hard ball. The symptoms of pain and stiffness that occur throughout the causal diagrams are believed to be the result of this process of blood thickening and becoming solid. It is the antithesis of the strong flow of blood required for good health.

The formation of a blood ball indicates that *miyet yawga* has reached a serious stage where palpitations, raised blood pressure, dizziness, blurriness and headaches become everyday occurrences. Tingling and numbness can also be present. Back pain followed by stiffness then occurs. The most serious symptom is stiffness in the neck that rises towards the head. This indicates that the solid ball of blood has moved progressively upwards from the stomach, causing stiffness locally on its journey, until it finally reaches the brain. The headaches, blurriness and dizziness thus constitute evidence of the blood ball moving out of the terrain of a menstrual illness and into the realm of a serious, possibly life threatening occurrence. The result of such an event is madness, shock, and sometimes death. Madness due to menstrual disorders comes in varying degrees including having an "unsound mind," or exhibiting "abnormal psychology," and finally there is madness itself.

Until recently the cure for irregular menstruation involved consulting an indigenous medical practitioner who would alter the diet. Remnants of this tradition are still practiced, but much of this knowledge has been lost or otherwise combined with a variety of treatments in the government traditional medicine training schools, hospitals, and clinics. For example, many women advocate eating pickled tea leaves (*lapeq*) and palm tree fruit to treat irregular menstruation. Conversely, eating sour foods, and sometimes hot, spicy food can lead to the staunching of blood flow.

At the Traditional Medicine Hospital, a majority of the female patients are diagnosed with "women's diseases." Dietary changes that include the Six Burmese Tastes (sweet, sour, hot, cold, salty, and bitter) are prescribed, as is an emmenagogue (Traditional Medicine Formula No. 15) (Aung Naing, n.d.). For example, in June, 1996, at the *Bohtataung* Traditional Medicine Clinic in Rangoon, a middle-aged woman with her white hair tied in a bun and wearing a cotton *longyi*[7] waits on the wooden bench to see the *Saya*.[8] Within a few minutes of history taking, the practitioner diagnoses the woman with menstrual dysfunction and Traditional Medicine Formula No. 15 is prescribed. The practitioner turns to me and explains that the formula consists of red and yellow sandalwood and cardamom. The practitioner diagnoses the woman's menstrual dysfunction as occurring around the time of her menopause, specifically due to anemia because "the flow of menstrual blood is not good."

The formula grown and pressed into powder at the Traditional Medicine Hospital is one of three emmenagogues prescribed depending upon the particular *miyet yawga* diagnosed. The composition of both commercial and official *thwe-ze* is a carefully guarded secret. Many families who harbor knowledge of indigenous medical practices have made and sold their own *thwe-ze* in their local area for several generations. *Thwe-ze* in Burma comes in an astonishing variety of types. The constant element is red sandalwood which gives *thwe-ze* its "hot" classification in the indigenous humoral system. Advertisements in magazines and newspapers promise secret ingredients of great potency. The following two vignettes give an indication of the range of beliefs about emmenagogue ingredients.

Vignette 2

My adopted daughter had irregular menstruation and then it stopped for six months and she became paler and paler. Pus came out from under her fingernails and then she died. She was twenty-two years old. She was treated by a traditional Burmese doctor at a private clinic.

What treatment did she have?

Medicine for "women's disease."

What are the ingredients?

It's a very expensive *thwe-ze: "chauq thwe."* It's a stone that you soak in water and the water becomes red. Also, the blood of a rhinoceros and parts of the horn.

In the next vignette, a biomedically-trained physician working in the relocated townships told me that:

Vignette 3

Another expensive *thwe-ze* is from a bird in Dawei. The bird is large and lives on the sea cliffs. The bird vomits up food that dries out and people collect it. People believe this will be in the *thwe-ze*, but I don't think so. You know what is really in *thwe-ze*? Corticosteroids. It's an illegal use for them. It's very dangerous. Even a university teacher, one of my friends, takes it every day. She developed blood blisters (like a pigment), like a bruise that doesn't disappear.

The humoral classificatory system common throughout many parts of the world, and especially in Southeast Asia (Foster, 1994), that creates distinctions between kinds of foods is maintained in contemporary Burma although the contents of such classifications differs markedly. The vignettes and in-depth interviews illustrate, however, that emmenagogues such as *thwe-ze* and injections of the contraceptive, *Depo-*

Provera,[9] have become the two main ways in which Burmese women attempt to manipulate their menstrual flow.

LIFE, DEATH, AND WEAKNESS IN BURMA'S PERI-URBAN TOWNSHIPS

Weakness

High living costs and indebtedness are the reasons that women in the relocated townships give for feeling unwell. This is usually characterized as weakness. *Thwe aah neh*[10] translates literally as weakness of the blood but it is often called anemia in Burma because of a perceived similarity of symptoms such as paleness. Weakness is a central idiom of distress (Nichter, 1981) in contemporary Burma. Inadequate economic resources lead inevitably to feelings of sadness and to constant worry. A consequence is an imbalance in the harmony that is required for health both within the body and between the body and the environment. White mucal discharge, either clotted (as in candidiasis) or viscous, is conceived of as red blood which has become pale and weak and is an indication of the body's lack of strength and thus ill health. It is thus commonly thought to be the first sign that weakness, sadness and fatigue are combining to cause irregular menstruation or a lack of menstruation. The ultimate solution to weakness and its more serious complication, irregular blood flow, is currently implausible. It involves rectifying the broader socioeconomic and political conditions that contribute to women worrying over finances, having many children they cannot feed, and relieving the general poverty that haunts the lives of most peri-urban township residents.

Abortion

Within the causal diagrams drawn by the women are a number of common themes such as childbirth, weakness, and amenorrhea. Abortion figures equally often and a great deal of cultural knowledge exists about varieties of abortion and miscarriages and ways to staunch hemorrhaging.

Women in the relocated townships are adamant that their decision to attempt to abort pregnancies stems from their impoverished situation and their inability to look after and to feed additional children. It is not a decision made lightly and they are aware of the danger of maternal death in their decision to seek illegal abortions. Many women initially deny knowledge of abortion because of its illegality. The focus group discussions included more than twenty ways of terminating pregnancies including jumping from heights, lifting heavy weights, pressure on the abdomen using a hot brick, and a variety of recipes that involve combinations of "hot foods." Before these methods are used, large amounts of *thwe-ze* are ingested because of its "hotness" and ability to create a strong blood flow.

Following abortions or deliberate miscarriages, women attempt to stop the flow of blood, as a too strong blood flow is believed to be as injurious as too little blood flow. Sometimes this becomes a life-threatening situation and women are admitted to local and city hospitals because of serious hemorrhaging. Several local hospitals are known as "green" hospitals because of the "green" or untimely, early deaths of so many patients. One particular hospital is greatly feared and people report seeing ghosts all around the hospital grounds. These ghosts are the souls of babies and mothers who have died in childbirth and as a consequence of illegal abortions.

The following two vignettes give an indication of the responses to questions about abortion.

Vignette 4

> I terminated my last pregnancy by using the *lethe* [traditional birth attendant]. She used a stick in the vagina. After that, I didn't have any further problems. If I hadn't terminated the pregnancy, my smallest child wouldn't have had enough breast milk. Also, I thought the pregnancy was only two months old, but it was really three months old. I was very unhappy that I didn't have enough money to have the baby, so I had to do [abort] it.

Vignette 5

> During our worst economic times, I was one month pregnant and I wanted to end it. So I drank four packets of *Kathypan [thwe-ze]* but it didn't work, and when the child was born, his skin was yellow. At seven months of age he became worse and we took him to the hospital. The doctors suggested that we go to Yangon [Rangoon] because they'd never seen that kind of problem before. But the problem was that we didn't have enough money to go [to Rangoon]. The child died at the [local] hospital.

A 1987 survey by UNICEF of 168 towns found that 52% of all registered maternal deaths in Burma were due to women attempting to procure abortions (UNICEF 1995:26). The large amount of knowledge about abortion methods and emergency situations resulting from abortion, coupled with the ease with which abortion was discussed in the surveys, suggests that the strong link between abortion, poverty, and maternal mortality continues to exist in the peri-urban townships (see Whittaker A. this volume). Not only does this link exist, but the women interviewed know that the "real" problem is not a medical one, but an economic one, and that economics is inextricably tied to the current political situation.

Several authors have demonstrated the use of menstrual regulators as abortifacients in areas where abortion is illegal (Sobo 1996; Nations et al. 1997; *Boston Globe* 1998; Whittaker 2000). Some of these authors have referred to a "hidden reproductive transcript," suggesting that these practices are a way of expressing collective public dissent at the policies and practices of the medical institutions controlled by the state (Nations et al. 1997; Whittaker 2000). Others argue that the ambiguity in definitions and semantics surrounding menstrual regulation, emmenagogues, purgatives, and abortifacients, allow "women flexibility in interpreting the meanings of their missed periods and the physical effects of the remedy" (Sobo 1996). This latter interpretation is closer to the situation in the peri-urban townships where abortion is not condoned within the community and has a long history in Burma. Resistance to the Burmese state via reproductive health practices is a very low priority for impoverished women who take very seriously their responsibilities to existing children and relatives and who generally must make pragmatic, rather than political, decisions.

Childbirth

There is a Burmese saying: "A woman in childbirth is like a man [going down a river] on a raft." Childbirth has long been acknowledged as a dangerous time for women, not just because of the risk of maternal death, but also because of the postpartum period (*me dwin*) when special care must be taken. The body is cold from blood loss and must be slowly reheated. Because resistance to illness is lowered at this time, new mothers must be insulated from shock or sudden change. The precautions taken in this period are also followed by women who have had complications in terminating pregnancies. They too seek to staunch the flow of blood and keep the body free from harm. Such postpartum beliefs and practices are common in Southeast Asia (Dixon 1993) and many Burmese women remain near a fire made from bamboo during the postpartum period. Washing of the hair is unacceptable as it cools the body, and heating rather than cooling foods are eaten at this time. In addition, foods that are thought to restrict blood flow (such as sour and bitter foods) are consumed in the *me dwin* period.

A common illness thought to result from the body becoming too cold in the postpartum period is *miyet kyan* which means a menstrual sickness whose main symptom is "chills."[11] The focus group discussions also included illnesses in the postpartum period caused by giving birth at the beginning of the monsoon season when several months of heavy rain led to an inability to stay dry and warm.[12] This emphasis upon chills, upon the body being excessively cooled, and the difficulties of staying dry are especially prominent concerns in the parts of the relocated townships that flood annually. Dirt roads become rivers of mud and earthen floors in many homes become quagmires. Several households I have visited have regular flooding of more than half a meter of water in their huts. They build their sleeping platforms as high as possible to remain above the water line during the monsoon period.

Childbirth is thus a time when new mothers must take good care of themselves through observing postpartum taboos, diet changes, and "heating" practices. In the townships this postpartum period is made more dangerous because of the difficulties of staying dry and warm and because of the additional burden of worry placed upon mothers that results from the bleak economic prospects of relocated residents.

MADNESS, MISERY, AND MENSTRUAL ILLNESS

At the beginning of the paper I described how a majority of people in the relocated townships are poor and unemployed. The women in the focus groups who are unemployed believe that their life will be the same, day after day. They have little hope that their lives will improve. Their hopes are that their children may escape the relocated townships and find a life where a steady income leads to possibilities denied to the current generation. For many people this hope is tinged with the sadness of losing their sense of place. For example, residents who have been relocated from the base of Mandalay Hill mourn the loss of the famous pagodas that ringed their township and especially the Mandalay Hill Pagoda that rose above them and was the central landmark by which they oriented their lives.

Smaller land allotments mean that extended families have been broken up with more nucleated family units becoming the norm. For older people this can mean living alone without any means of financial income other than donations from well wishing neighbors and friends. For women with many children, smaller households mean less family support and childcare and that the husband generally becomes the primary income earner. Domestic violence, sexual bartering, incest and child abuse occur more frequently when the regular checks and balances of extended family living are no longer possible. These social problems are aggravated by the tensions of unemployment and underemployment.

In times of continual worry and unhappiness, madness is always a possibility. Women at the Rangoon Psychiatric Hospital often describe their behavior prior to admission as: "I was mad at the time." Events and illnesses threaten the balance that exists within the body and between the body and the world. Often these imbalances can be corrected by extra care, a certain diet, or recourse to indigenous medical practitioners or biomedical interventions. Thus "women's diseases" in Burma are common, multi-causal and can usually be cured. "Women's diseases" can lead to madness and death when they occur in the midst of an already unhealthy situation. This is why peri-urban women believe that being relocated has put them at risk of illness. A female patient at the Rangoon Psychiatric Hospital explained to me the preconditions for potential madness in the following way.

Vignette 6

> I was eighteen when I got married. Just after my marriage was a happy time. After my baby was born, though, I suffered from many illnesses. I had irregular menstruation after the delivery so I had an injection of *Depo-Provera*. I went to many traditional Burmese doctors and many western hospitals. After that I stopped the injections and I had no menstruation for a year. I took traditional medicines that I swallowed and I also used lotions.

Why did you stop going to traditional healers?

I thought I wasn't improving . . .

The physician in charge of the patient interrupts with:

We think she has neurosis because she's always worrying about her child and herself.

I ask the patient: Do you think you have a mental illness?

I don't think it's a problem coming from the mind. I think it's because of the irregularity of my menstrual cycle.

What happens if you don't menstruate?

Skin eruptions, backache, and pain in the mouth. I don't think I'll go mad from this *miyet yawga*, but if my husband gets into trouble, maybe I will. If he can't work very much, I think I'll go mad. My parents-in-law have already come to us asking for money to repair their house, to buy food, for many reasons . . .

Madness, as this woman's vignette demonstrates, is rarely caused by one incident alone. Grief, loneliness, and other vicissitudes of everyday life can be borne with community and family support. Buddhism, in particular, provides a framework for understanding suffering and sorrow. There are many forms of traditional social organization and community support groups, both Buddhist and secular, that people can turn to in times of economic or other calamity. In the relocated townships, many of these structures have broken down, or have been infiltrated and suborned by the military government. The threat of madness thus figures more acutely in the thoughts of women of peri-urban townships because there are fewer support networks that may ward off madness. More importantly, the socioeconomic situation of many of the peri-urban township residents is perilous and it is this combination of extreme economic vulnerability with the vicissitudes of quotidian life that allows the threat of madness to stalk the peri-urban townships.

POVERTY AND POLITICS

Many of the residents speak with great sorrow about the loss of their former neighborhoods and the move to the New Fields is given as a key reason for the general ill health of the majority of people in the townships. Economic hardship has resulted in malnutrition on a wide scale. Family land plots are small, necessitating the breaking up of extended family groups. I have met many families who live on a bamboo platform and cook and defecate in the mud below the platform. The monsoon rains transform the relocated townships into a sea of mud and diseases of poor sanitation are rife. Diarrhea, cholera epidemics, tuberculosis, polio, leprosy and physical and intellectual disabilities are common.

It is hard to find unmarried women in the townships. It is sheer economic necessity that requires women to re-marry as quickly as possible after divorce, abandonment, or widowhood. It is not surprising in this economic nightmare to find women agonizing over unplanned pregnancies, unemployment, rising debt levels and abandonment by their spouses. Prostitution occurs among young women living with their parents, abandoned, widowed or divorced women who have not yet remarried, as well as married women whose impoverished status necessitates the married couple agreeing that the woman will engage in prostitution until household finances improve. This latter situation occurs most often when husbands become disabled or ill or are unable to find employment. Almost the only women to be profiting in the relocated townships are women working in prostitution, women recruiting for prostitution rings, and women working as creditors with lending rates of over 30% per month. In interviews with over fifty women working in prostitution in Rangoon's peri-urban townships, the general consensus was that at any one time, one-third of all women of reproductive age in the peri-urban townships are engaged in prostitution.

As the townships become established, land speculation sometimes occurs. Remaining city residents begin buying land in the New Fields because of the increasing costs of urban living and in anticipation of being forcibly relocated in the coming years. The Burmese government, devoid of cash, often pays its employees in kind. This includes rice and oil but can also mean land in the relocated townships. This means that a group of "non-poor" residents exist. In one such newly established household I saw a large old television and an electric fan. This is the only house I have seen with such luxuries, apart from brothels and the houses of women who own brothels. No statistics are available because of the diverse socioeconomic groupings of different townships and wards within townships. For example, Mandalay's peri-urban townships contain both the most affluent and the most impoverished residents. Some sectors of the townships will have piped water and may have electricity, while others contain thatched huts or sleeping platforms with no facilities at all.

A small group of people within the townships (primarily government employees, brothel owners, and creditors) are not impoverished and perhaps this number will rise as more city residents seek cheaper land prices and as peri-urban infrastructure and small businesses become established. The relocated townships are only a few kilometers from the main cities and better transportation links will continue to make them viable alternatives to the escalating costs of city living. This small group contrasts markedly, however, with the daily intake into the feeding centers of children dying from malnutrition, dehydration, and preventable diseases such as measles and of women presenting to hospitals bleeding to death from incomplete abortions. The incongruity of these various groups of people living side by side can only be understood within the wider framework of a military dictatorship intent upon suppressing potential democratic neighborhoods and creating new urban centers that immortalize the role of the military in Burmese society.

CONCLUSION

The focus group discussions and individual interviews with women of reproductive age in the relocated townships have taken a full week of long days, beginning before the heat starts and ending with the brief Burmese twilight. I put down my pen and glance out the open doorway. The women helping me have found a thin red cow and are paying the owner for some fresh milk that they take turns drinking from the bucket. My skin and clothes are coated with a fine layer of red dust. It looks like I have been doused with a packet of *thwe-ze*. The women are beginning to disperse to their bamboo huts, calling to their children, some of whom are climbing nearby trees and tormenting small insects with broken-off branches. As the evening shadows lengthen I begin the journey back into town. I pass dusty laborers returning from construction sites. As there is no electricity in much of the townships, most women will be cooking rice on an open fire. There is little entertainment in these peri-urban townships. The sound of guitars is not common here as it is in the more established townships.

The women have painted a bleak picture of their hopes and aspirations and have described days filled with the same constant frustrations and worries. It has been my aim in this paper to show how the women link their reproductive health with their local environment, their socio-economic situation, and the amoral economy of a military dictatorship that has created impoverished slums in which illegal abortions, hunger, and worry are everyday occurrences. Burmese conceptions of pathophysiology link together all these elements of everyday life and create an embodied account of contemporary life in the peri-urban townships.

NOTES

1. In this paper I use the pre-1989 names for Yangon (Rangoon) and the Union of Myanmar (Burma). I use the term "Burmans" to refer to the ethnic majority group and "Burmese" to designate all those who live within Burma's boundaries.

2. Qualitative, quantitative, and existing data was collected and triangulated. Data collection used a combination of Rapid Assessment Procedures (RAPs), questionnaires, key informant and in-depth interviews, and Participatory Learning and Activity techniques (PLAs) (Jayakaran 1996). Each of the mothers in the sample has at least one child under five years of age and was recruited on a voluntary basis. Cluster sampling was used in the study so as to accurately represent the population density in each ward of each township. Many women in the study volunteered information about the number of abortions they had sought, but no women admitted to being involved in casual sex work.

3. In 1994 and 1996-7 this included fieldwork at the Traditional Medicine Hospital in Rangoon, and several outpatient clinics in surrounding townships (and several visits to the Traditional Medicine Hospital in Mandalay). During this period I also worked at the Rangoon Psychiatric Hospital and more generally in the peri-urban townships of Rangoon and Mandalay. Midwives, traditional medicine practitioners, community healers (*yankus*), local health officials, and sex workers participated in the study. Some of the conclusions of the earlier studies are included in this paper.

4. Disease has a direct translation in Burmese, but there is no Burmese word for either illness or sickness.

5. *Thwe-ze* is one of the three traditional pharmacopoeias that were the staple of Burmese medicine cabinets (along with *lei-ze* and *yeq-ze*). The Burmese medical tradition in which *thwe-ze* is situated has disintegrated since the time of British colonization (Government of Burma 1951). It is now practiced by few Burmese in the form that reached its most comprehensive zenith prior to the nineteenth century, apart from its altered form in the official traditional medicine sector.

6. All names are pseudonyms.

7. A *longyi* consists of two meters of material sewn together to form a tube of fabric which is wrapped tightly around the waist. A piece of black fabric is sewn onto the top border of the *longyi* that is twisted and tucked into the *longyi* to ensure that it doesn't fall down.

8. *Saya* means "teacher" or "master." It can be applied to almost any trade or profession. In this case it refers to an indigenous medicine practitioner, known as a *sae* [medicine] *saya.*

9. Interestingly, oral contraceptives are believed to be a cause of irregular menstruation (and this could be true if they are not taken correctly), but contraceptive injections are most often believed to ensure regular menstruation. It is possible that twenty-one day contraceptive packs may be used by women continuously so that menstruation cannot occur in the fourth week. This is complicated by the fact that a small number of women cite *Depo-Provera* injections as a reason for the cessation of menstruation. Injections are viewed as rendering miraculous, almost spontaneous, cures (see Skidmore 1998 for a discussion of "the magic of needles" in Burma).

10. "Weakness" is used across many domains of everyday life. It has multiple causes. It is, perhaps, the reason that vitamin injections, especially vitamin B injections, are often the first recourse when individuals feel unwell. It is an inexpensive quick fix. Problems arise when the vitamins are a long way past their expiration date and through the reuse of syringes and their improper sterilization. As few people who administer injections are trained in the correct procedure, abscesses and other venous problems and infections also occur.

11. All of the "cooling" illnesses placed in this category are more likely to occur in women who are overweight. Particularly in rural Burma, the successful cessation of the postpartum period is marked by a celebration (*me tweq teh*) which translates as "leaving the fire."

12. Washing the body and particularly the use of soap was reported as a cause of *miyet yawga*. Joint pain in the extremities is also grouped under the rubric of "women's diseases" if it appears to occur in conjunction with symptoms related to blood flow.

REFERENCES

Aung Naing (ed.) (n.d.). *Myanmar Traditional Medicine: Manual for Health Basic Training Course.* Yangon: The Union of Myanmar, State Traditional Medicinal Council.

Boston Globe (1988). Pills and Parallels. *Boston Globe.* Boston, MA, Oct. 6., p. 20.

Buck-Morss, S. (1989). *Dialectics of Seeing: Walter Benjamin and the Arcades Project.* Cambridge and London: MIT Press.

Dixon, G. (1993). Ethnicity and Infant Mortality in Malaysia. *Asia-Pacific Population Journal.* 8(2), 23-54.

Farmer, P. (1992). *AIDS and Accusation: Haiti and the Geography of Blame.* Berkeley: University of California Press.

Foster, G.M. (1994). *Hippocrates' Latin American Legacy. Humoral Medicine in the Third World.* Langhome: Gordon and Breach Science Publishers.

Good, B. (1977). The Heart of What's the Matter: The Semantics of Illness in Iran. *Culture, Medicine and Psychiatry.* 1(1), 25-58.

Government of Burma (1951). (RCE) *Report of the Committee of Enquiry into the Indigenous System of Medicine.* Rangoon: Superintendent, Government Printing and Stationery.

Jayakaran, R. (1996). *Participatory Learning and Action.* Madras: World Vision India.

Kulczycki, A., Potts, M. and A. Rosefield (1996). Abortion and Fertility Regulation. *The Lancet.* 347(9016), 1663-1669.

Nations, M.K., Misago, C. and W. Fonseca (1997). Women's Hidden Transcripts About Abortion in Brazil. *Social Science and Medicine.* 44(12), 1833-1845.

Nichter, M. (1981). Idioms of Distress, Alternatives in the Expression of Psychosocial Distress: A Case Study from South India. *Culture, Medicine and Psychiatry.* 5, 379-408.

Singh, S. (1998). Adolescent Childbearing in Developing Countries: A Global Review. *Studies in Family Planning.* 29(2), 117-137.

Skidmore, M. (1998). *Flying Through a Skyful of Lies: Survival Strategies and the Politics of Fear in Urban Myanmar (Burma).* Unpublished Ph.D. Thesis. Montreal: McGill University.

Sobo, E.J. (1996). Abortion Traditions in Rural Jamaica. *Social Science and Medicine.* 42(4), 495-508.

UNICEF (1995). *Children and Women in Myanmar: A Situation Analysis.* Yangon: Myanmar.

Van der Walle, E. (1997). Flowers and Fruits: Two Thousand Years of Menstrual Regulation. *The Journal of Interdisciplinary History.* 28(2), 183-203.

Whittaker, A.M. (2000). *Intimate Knowledge: Women and Their Health in North-East Thailand.* Sydney: Allen and Unwin.

Reproducing Inequalities:
Abortion Policy and Practice in Thailand

Andrea Whittaker, PhD

SUMMARY. Abortion is illegal in Thailand, except in cases when it is considered necessary for a woman's health or in the case of rape. Yet abortions remain common and an important public health issue for women in Thailand. Based upon eight months' ethnographic research carried out in Northeast Thailand, this paper presents findings from a survey of 164 women of reproductive age in rural villages and from interviews with 19 women who have had illegal abortions. A range of techniques to induce abortions are used, including the consumption of abortifacients, massage, and uterine injections by untrained practitioners, and procedures carried out by trained medical personnel. This paper examines the effects of the current laws through the experiences of women who have undergone illegal abortions. Within the restrictive legal context, risk is stratified along economic lines. Poorer women have

Andrea Whittaker is Joint Lecturer, Key Center for Women's Health in Society and the Melbourne Institute of Asian Languages and Societies, The University of Melbourne, Melbourne, Victoria, 3010, Australia (E-mail: a.whittaker@unimelb.edu.au).

The author wishes to thank the women who generously shared their stories. The author also wishes to thank the Thai National Research Council for permission to conduct this research. The author offers many thanks to Amornrat Sricamsuk of the Faculty of Nursing, Khon Kaen University who worked as a research assistant on this project and to her family for their hospitality. In addition, the author thanks the staff of the Faculty of Nursing, Khon Kaen University for their continued support, and to Peter Ross and Bruce Missingham of the Australian National University who assisted with the translations in this paper.

This research was funded by an Australian Research Council (ARC) Postdoctoral Fellowship and ARC Large Grant.

[Haworth co-indexing entry note]: "Reproducing Inequalities: Abortion Policy and Practice in Thailand." Whittaker, Andrea. Co-published simultaneously in *Women & Health* (The Haworth Medical Press, an imprint of The Haworth Press, Inc.) Vol. 35, No. 4, 2002, pp. 101-119; and: *Women's Health in Mainland Southeast Asia* (ed: Andrea Whittaker) The Haworth Medical Press, an imprint of The Haworth Press, Inc., 2002, pp. 101-119. Single or multiple copies of this article are available for a fee from The Haworth Document Delivery Service [1-800-HAWORTH, 9:00 a.m. - 5:00 p.m. (EST). E-mail address: getinfo@haworthpressinc.com].

101

little choice but to resort to abortions by untrained practitioners. There is evidence of wide public support for the reform of the abortion laws to widen the circumstances under which abortion is legal. An ongoing movement, led by women's groups, medical and legal professionals, seeks to reform the law. *[Article copies available for a fee from The Haworth Document Delivery Service: 1-800-HAWORTH. E-mail address: <getinfo@ haworthpressinc.com> Website: <http://www.HaworthPress.com> © 2002 by The Haworth Press, Inc. All rights reserved.]*

KEYWORDS. Abortion, Thailand, qualitative methods, legal status

What can we do? The law of our own homeland, they've made it like this . . . When it's soft, it's too soft. When it is tough, it is too tough . . . (Female participant in a rural focus group discussion 1998)

In Thailand, women wishing to terminate an unplanned pregnancy are left with little choice but to have an illegal abortion. Under section 305 of the Criminal Code of 1957, abortion is illegal in Thailand under all circumstances except if necessary for a woman's health[1] or in the case of reported rape or seduction of a girl under fifteen. Despite the illegal status of abortion, and comprehensive access to family planning, it is estimated that approximately 80,000 to 300,000 illegal induced abortions are performed throughout the country annually (Chaturachinda et al. 1981; Ladipo 1989; Narkavonnakit and Bennett 1981; Thailand 1990). This paper highlights the effects of the current restrictive laws through the experiences of women who have undergone illegal abortions (see also Skidmore this volume). Although wealthy women can access safe terminations by trained personnel in clean conditions, such procedures are expensive. Poor women attempt to self-abort, and failing that, risk abortions conducted by untrained personnel. An ongoing effort to reform the abortion laws continues, led by women's groups, medical and legal professionals.

Women's access to abortion in Thailand remains a major public health issue, but also reflects the inequalities of Thai society, for it is poor women who are most affected by the legal restrictions.

STUDIES OF ABORTION IN THAILAND

The majority of research on the issue in Thailand occurred during the late 1970s and early 1980s, coinciding with unsuccessful attempts to liberalize the abortion laws. These studies provided important public health information documenting the incidence of illegal abortions, morbidity and mortality, characteristics of women who abort, correlations with contraceptive use and family planning, and the practices and characteristics of abortion practitioners (see Chaturachinda et al. 1981; Koetsawang et al. 1978; Pinchun and Chullapram 1993; Pongthai et al. 1984; Rattakul 1971; Rauyajin 1979; Thailand 1984; Toongsuwan et al. 1973).

Recent studies confirm the impact of abortion as a major source of morbidity and mortality for women in Thailand. A 1993 study of 968 cases of illegal abortions in five provincial hospitals found 1% (13 women) died due to subsequent complications. Heavy bleeding was reported in 13% of the total cases. Hysterectomy to remove a severely infected or perforated uterus was performed in 22 women and a blood transfusion was required in 104 women (10.7%) (Koetsawang 1993). Ministry of Public Health Statistics report 40 deaths from abortion across the country in 1991 (Thailand 1993:147). Twenty-eight maternal deaths caused by abortion were recorded in 1992 and 14 deaths were recorded in 1994.[2] A widely cited 1980 survey of illegal abortion in the poor rural Northeast province of Chaiyaphum found that one tenth of the women who had abortions by untrained practitioners experienced complications serious enough to require hospitalization, while 25% of them experienced some form of complication and morbidity but did not seek hospital care (Narkavonnakit and Bennett 1981:60). The same study calculated an abortion rate of 107 per 1,000 rural women age 15-44, or 160 per 1,000 married rural women, compared to a marital fertility rate for the same province at that time of 190 per 1,000 women (Narkavonnakit and Bennett 1981). That high estimate was calculated from interviews with abortionists to estimate caseloads in the province, rather than the more usual technique of extrapolation from complications presenting to hospitals. No more recent studies have been conducted using the same techniques. It is unlikely that such a high rate still exists in rural areas given the now extensive family planning coverage, but it does highlight the need for understanding abortion in rural communities.

The most recent epidemiological study of abortion in Thailand is a WHO funded study conducted in 1999 of clients of public hospitals in 76 provinces by the Ministry of Public Health (Boonthai and Warakamin 2001). It included cross sectional data collection of a total of 45,990 cases of women presenting with symptoms relating to spontaneous miscarriage or abortion, of whom 28.5% were found to have had induced abortions (19.54 per 1,000 live births). The main serious complication was septicemia with 14 deaths (0.11%). Interviews with a selected sample of 4,588 of the women found that the main reasons for inducing an abortion were socioeconomic problems (56.8%) and family planning difficulties, such as pregnancy at an inappropriate age, pregnancies too close together or unplanned pregnancies after having achieved desired family size (34.4%). The methods used to induce abortions included injection or insertion of substances into the vaginal canal (40.6%), vaginal suppository (13.6%), oral tablets (11.6%), and massage (11%). About 12% of these women had tried to induce their abortions themselves, and 40% had serious complications such as severe hemorrhage (11.8%), septicemia (12.4%), pelvic inflammatory disease (12.0%), and uterine perforation (7.4%). The authors of the study call for the revision of abortion laws to allow women access to safer methods of induced abortion, and highlight the need for improved public health programs to prevent unplanned pregnancies.

METHODS

As most studies on abortion in Thailand have been demographic or epidemiological studies, there remains little known about the experiences and point of view of women who abort (an exception is Kanokwan 2000). This paper is based upon eight months' fieldwork in rural Northeast Thailand in 1997-1998. The aim of the research was to study cultural and social issues relating to women's access to abortion services, their experiences and perceptions, and to understand the broader political context of abortion debate in Thailand. The impetus for this research was derived from my previous experience studying women's health in a long-term ethnographic study in a rural village from 1991-1993 (see Whittaker 2000).

Anthropological techniques are well-suited to gathering the rich personal detail I wished to obtain for this study (Huntington et al. 1993). For example, Bleek's study on abortion in rural Ghana found that the information obtained through surveys was less reliable than the data he obtained through long-term fieldwork and familiarity with the community (Bleek 1987:319). The study was designed using a variety of techniques in order to enhance the reliability and validity of data on such a socially sensitive topic (see Coeytaux et al. 1989; Helitzer-Allen et al. 1994). The complete study included 173 structured interviews in a survey of women of reproductive age in four randomly selected rural districts, seven focus group discussions, and 19 case studies of women who had recent illegal abortions. All interviews were conducted in the local Isan/Lao dialect by me and a trained local research assistant.

The setting of this study, Northeast Thailand, is the least developed and poorest region of Thailand, with the highest incidence of poverty, calculated at 37.4% of the population in 1987/89 (Phongpaichit and Baker 1995:65). Most villagers in the region are rice-farmers, supplementing their meager incomes by periods of migration for work in urban centers.

CHARACTERISTICS OF WOMEN WHO ABORT

The common assumption in Thai media reports is that unplanned pregnancies and abortion are problems of young, unmarried women. However, studies of abortion in Thailand report that 75% of women who seek abortions are married and primarily motivated by economic or family reasons (Koetsawang 1993). Boonthai and Warakamin (2001) found that 30% of women presenting to hospitals with complications from induced abortion in 1999 were less than 20 years of age.

Despite the high use of contraceptives in Thailand, unplanned pregnancies remain a common dilemma for women. The contraceptive pill, injectables, IUDs, condoms and now Norplant are widely accessible at government clinics. According to the National Statistical Office in 1997, the contraceptive prevalence rate for married women of reproductive age 15-44 was 75.2%. The contraceptive pill is the most popular form of contraception used by married couples (28.4%), with female sterilization ranked second (23.9%) (Rabiabloke and Wilairat 1998). A recent study of 80 women with unplanned pregnancies suggests that many married women experience unplanned pregnancies despite using modern contraceptives. They fell pregnant after they experienced difficulty with their contraceptives, either using them incorrectly, discontinuing their use due to side effects, or experiencing contraceptive failure (Kanokwan 2000). The same study found unmarried women have limited access to contraceptives as it is assumed that they are not sexually active and "contraception is for married people" (Kanokwan 2000:11). Unmarried women tend to have limited knowledge about contraception and tend to depend upon condoms and other methods with high failure rates, such as counting days and withdrawal.

My research confirms this picture (Whittaker 2000). In the survey sample of 164 predominantly married rural women between the ages of

15 and 45 years,[3] 41 (24%) had ever experienced unplanned pregnancies and 11% had an unplanned pregnancy while using a contraceptive. Many of these women had experienced problems with their IUDs or had missed taking the pill. Of the 41 women who had experienced unplanned pregnancies, 23 took no action and continued the pregnancy. The other 18 women (11%) attempted abortions through various means, some successfully, some not.

Elsewhere I have written in detail of the factors influencing women's decisions to abort. Most women said that their inability to afford to raise another child due to poor economic circumstances was their main motivation to attempt to abort the pregnancy (Whittaker 2001). The circumstances that shape couples' reproductive decisions are complex and include the effects of poverty and economic inequalities, the configurations and expectations of gender relations, meanings of motherhood and nurturance, the changing position of women, shifting lifestyle expectations, and the changing value of children. Although women are aware of the illegality of abortion, the law has little perceived relevance to the realities of villagers' lives.

WOMEN'S STORIES

The stories of women who have had illegal abortions force us to confront its realities. Women speak of their fear as they contemplate the risks, the pain of repeated attempts, the relief and regrets that accompany the abortion. In order to illustrate the constraints that current laws place on women and the risks that poorer women face, I present two stories. In the first, Nang Su tells of her attempts to self-induce her abortion, and her resort to untrained practitioners. In the second, Nang Oi tells of her experience in the safer environment of a private hospital. While her abortion is described as less painful and less dangerous, the secrecy, the expense, the overcrowding and lack of privacy in the wards, are all consequences of the illegality of abortion.

Case One: Nang Su

Nang Su lives in a rural village in Roi Et province. She is 30 years old. She is married to A Et and they have three sons, ages 15, 12 and 7. They live together with her mother and an orphaned nephew. They are rice farmers with 20 rai of farm land (1 rai equals 0.16 ha). Her eldest son has left school and makes a little extra income from caring for cattle. About four months before this interview she had an abortion. She was two months pregnant. She has used contraceptive pills for seven years since the birth of her last son.

> I'd been taking them for a month, then later on, [I thought] 'Here, I've been taking a lot of tablets,' so I spread them out a bit. It's not that I skipped a lot at all. I skipped a single tablet. Two tablets, one, something like that. Like it was a mistake. So the child was conceived . . .

She confirmed her pregnancy with a urine test at the local primary health station. She was very worried to find out she was pregnant. Like many poor rural women she did not feel she could raise another child, with all the effort, expense and lost opportunities for her family that another child would represent.

> I have a lot of children already, and I am old already, I wasn't able to look after it . . . My thoughts went everywhere. I was worried that I was pregnant. I was scared. I was afraid . . . Oh, all a blur, I was afraid it wouldn't come out. Afraid of all sorts of things, right. Well I consulted with one friend. I asked her. Afraid of having a child, right. Who wants to [have an abortion]? I am a mother! We discussed it. We talked together.

Nang Su's story is a typical one in that she first attempted an abortion through use of an emmenagogue. These are marketed in drug stores throughout Thailand as *ya satri*[1] or "women's medicines." They are defined as humorally "hot" medicines, sometimes also called *ya dong* (pickled medicines). Sixteen percent of 164 village women interviewed in this study had used some form of emmenagogue at some time to regulate their menstruation. Other drugs such as aspirin in alcohol, *Kano* (500 mg tetracycline), various hormonal regulators, and the contraceptive pill are also commonly consumed by women in their abortion attempts.

After an unsuccessful attempt at self-inducing an abortion, Nang Su went to see a massage abortionist who is well known in her village. In the 1980 survey of abortion in the rural province of Chaiyaphum mentioned above, the majority (60%) of rural abortions were induced by massage (Narkavonnakit and Bennett 1981:60). Massage abortions involve locating the foetal mass by external palpation and then using a pressing, pulling and jabbing motion with the fingers to dislodge it.

Women often undergo this procedure several times until they start bleeding. Many women then present to their local District Hospital once the abortion is inevitable, although for some, fear of discovery means that they do not seek care at all. Nang Su describes the procedure vividly.

> She squeezed for a long time. Loooong time!

> *How many hours, auntie?*

> Round about two hours . . . Squeezed till it hurt. Squeezed the uterus till it hurt. She *poked* like this. Poked altogether I reckon two hours.

> *What did you do?*

> I lay down with my knees up, right? Knees up like this. And [she] thrust down like this. Thrust down until it was over . . . In our village lots of people go [to the massage abortionist]. Now, we reckon that the little ones [the embryos] are getting more stubborn. They won't let them[selves] be poked away too easily. It'd come out with difficulty. E Siwi [another woman in the village] went repeatedly, all up three times [before her abortion was successful].

Nang Su's attempted massage abortion was unsuccessful. She describes the pregnancy as "stubborn." Accompanied by her husband, Nang Su went to the village of Ban Nang Long where she was given an injection per vagina. They paid 600 baht ($US12, the equivalent of over one week's pay) for the procedure. Injection abortions involve either a large syringe, urine catheter or a plastic tube inserted into the uterus. Any one of a range of substances are then injected, including saline, distilled water, cumin mixed with water, glucose, Dettol, alcohol, gasoline, Piton-S (an oxytocin drug) or Duogynon-Forte. Clearly, this is a highly dangerous procedure and injection abortions are over-represented in figures of hospitalized abortion cases, suggesting that this practice is one of the most harmful techniques used (Narkavonnakit and Bennett 1981).

> It was an ordinary house. The wife of an old village headman. She did it at her place. She did it downstairs in the kitchen . . . It was a syringe. They had you lie down, legs apart. They would take their

things and bring them themselves, put in the syringe [into the vagina] themselves. But when she had injected the medicine, then I was drowsy, reacting to the medicine.

After one day, Nang Su started to miscarry and the bleeding lasted for three days.

Fever! I was shaking. Almost like I was going to die there, all over . . . I was like this until they [a friend, probably a local injectionist] gave me a saline infusion. Like I was feverish and cold. At the time I went and boiled some water for a bath. It was then the blood came . . .

My body was cold, it was shaking all over. So I went to boil some water for a bath. The blood came then. My friend was able to give me some saline. Sitting like this the blood flowed out like that. It came out fairly strongly but gradually for quite a while. I was so cold. I had chills. She [the abortionist] had told me that I would have chills and all. Be all feverish. 'Don't be afraid at all. You'll have this sort of condition,' she told me . . . Oh, two, three days, then it stopped. It came out till I was afraid that all my blood would be gone.

Despite the fever and heavy bleeding Nang Su decided not to go to see a doctor. She told us she was still feeling weak but has recovered. She is now using Depo-Provera injections. Although she dislikes its side effects, she is reassured that she won't experience another unplanned pregnancy.

Case Two: Nang Oi

Nang Oi is 45 years old. She is married and has two daughters, 20 and 14 years old, who are both still living at home. She is also from a poor family with 25 rai of rice land. However, her family benefits from the income of her married daughter and husband who migrate regularly to Bangkok to work. The year before, in February, she aborted a third pregnancy. She wasn't using any method of birth control at that time as she thought she was too old to conceive. When she didn't menstruate she thought it was just natural for a woman of her age. Only when her breasts began to be full did she seek a doctor's advice and discovered that she was pregnant. She consulted with her partner who stated that it was her decision. It took her over two weeks to decide to have an abortion.

In contrast to Nang Su's experience, Nang Oi went to Bangkok where her younger sister lived and attended a private hospital there.

> I'd been for a check already. I was thinking pretty deeply there. For a long time it went on like that. It was no good thinking this and thinking that. At about two months, I was thinking this, thinking that. [By the time I decided I was] two and a half months pregnant. [If I had decided] at two months I probably could've gone and done it [easier] . . .

> I'm old, not young and strong any more. There's no way I'd be able to raise it . . . It was like, I'm at an age at which I have to be responsible. We're not able to raise a child. What can we do? We have to be stoic. [Before I went] I was thinking 'How will it be?' [I was] thinking about being with the doctor. [I said to myself] 'It will probably be fine, once I'm there with the doctor already.'

She found out about the hospital through her younger sister. Upon arrival at the hospital, she underwent an examination and brief counselling. She felt the doctors treated her well, speaking politely to her. After an ultrasound to confirm the gestation of the pregnancy, she was directed to a crowded ward and put on a drip.

> They didn't inject me. They gave it to me by way of the saline drip. Once the saline and the medicine had gone in, I had symptoms of stomach pains straight away. Then it was just one lump. It was just the same as giving birth to a child . . .

> They gave me the drip [from] about one o'clock till not quite six o'clock in the evening. But at that time, well, I was in pain and I didn't really look at the clock. But when I'd finished giving birth, right, I had finished giving birth, I looked at the clock and it wasn't yet six o'clock. We called the doctor over to look. The doctor came to look, they did some business for me, they put on a sanitary pad, and then I slept comfortably . . .

> I gave birth just the same as I'd give birth to a child . . . Lay down on a bed and gave birth there on the bed itself. Gave birth. And sometimes you could see kids, they were crying, I wasn't alone.

From time to time people would come in. There were a lot of people. They had nurses. But the doctors, they did their work. They saw I was old and thought I would faint. I was giving birth, wasn't I? They said 'Young people can't beat the old ones!' But they looked after me. Once they had gotten the body to come out, a child came out, see. But it wasn't very big, quite small, just over two months. When it had come out the pain went away just like giving birth to a child. They had me lay in at the hospital for a night. After that, I got up really early, and then slept straight away. Then about midday, my relatives came to get me.

The hospital was crowded with women. 'They sent them to the second floor, the third floor, and the fourth floor. [It was] full and overflowing'. . . . In her ward there were a number of young women, some of whom were having very late term abortions up to six months gestation. With no partitions or curtains between the beds the women could all see one another.

When I went, the students, they got them to lie on a bed, a patient's bed and they talked together. When they had stomach pains, they talked together. They'd say, '*I've* been here lots of times already.' They came from the [other clinic] together. They refer them there. It was a real pity, they're just the same, they were really in pain. If you're many months pregnant, it hurts a lot. I've given birth before, haven't I? These kids, they've never given birth. They don't know pain. They tend to cry out. But the doctors, they'd talk like this: 'It'll be over soon.' . . . In the room, [there were] two people to a bed. In that room there were about 20 beds.

The abortion was expensive, costing Nang Oi 5,000 baht (approx. $US100), the equivalent of many months' rural wages. "They charge 2,000 baht a month [gestation]. For two and a half months they charge 5,000 baht. For some people it was 10,000 for 5 months, 6 months it was 12,000."

Most rural women cannot afford such procedures, or else have difficulty accessing them. Although both Nang Su and Nang Oi are from poor rural families, Nang Oi has more access to disposable income through the wages of her eldest daughter and son-in law. This meant that she was able to afford a safer abortion in a private hospital setting. With a young family with no such resources, Nang Su had little choice but to use cheaper but more risky local untrained practitioners. In such ways, within the restrictive legal context, risk is stratified along economic lines.

The private clinics offering abortion services are occasionally subject to police raids. The illegality means services in clinics are often rushed and offer little follow-up care for women. Nang Oi describes her experience as "comfortable" and was reassured by the safety of the private hospital, "I feel they had good treatment. The kids or whoever, if they go they guarantee safety [for them]." However, the conditions she describes of overcrowded beds filled with women in pain seeing each other abort suggests the quality of care is poor.

Nang Oi has no regrets over her action:

> I've been to do it, there. I feel that, we don't have any obligation to feel anxious over that child. I won't have to worry about lots of different things. I won't have to raise the child, anything like that. We're this old already, right. We could raise them but not well enough. Now, I don't think [about it] any more. I don't have to think any more. I just think that they were born just thus far and I'll let it go according to karma (*kam*) right. Some people, they say to make merit [to reduce the demerit].

Nang Oi is still not practicing any form of contraception. When I expressed fear that she may fall pregnant again, she said that she was told it would be unlikely that she could fall pregnant again at her age. Her only fear is that her abortion might lead to the development of cancer that is understood to develop from the lack of cleanliness and disruption of the womb caused by an abortion (see Boonmongkon et al. this volume).

SOCIAL ACCEPTABILITY OF ABORTION

The numbers of women seeking abortions indicate that state morality as codified in Thai law is inconsistent with the realities women face in controlling their fertility. There is considerable evidence that the laws also fail to reflect Thai public attitudes towards abortion and the diverse ways in which the morality of abortion is negotiated in Thai society (Whittaker 2002). Among the villagers I interviewed, abortion is considered to be a life-destroying act that constitutes a serious Buddhist sin/demerit. It carries karmic consequences not only for the mother who will be reincarnated into a less auspicious life, but also for the aborted fetus that is understood to have missed an opportunity to be reincarnated to improve its karmic status. Many women cited fear of *bap* (Buddhist demerit) as the reason why they chose to continue with an unplanned pregnancy. Late term abortions are considered to involve greater demerit than earlier term abortions. In Thai Buddhism, unlike in Japan, there is no memorial rite for an aborted fetus (see Hardacre 1997). Instead, women such as Nang Oi describe making merit (*tham bun*) and giving alms to the monks as means of minimizing the bad karmic consequences of their act. They speak of "washing away the sin" (*lang bap*) referring to the ritual of pouring water during temple services as a libation to transfer the merit acquired to the dead. Some women also suggested that observing extra Buddhist precepts as a lay person or during brief periods ordained as a nun may assist in minimizing the level of demerit.

In a review of Buddhist views on abortion, bioethicist Pinit Ratanakul suggests that although institutionalized Buddhism rejects abortion, most lay Thai Buddhists agree with a middle path on the morality of abortion: "a way that avoids the two extremes of laxity and rigidity in the observance of the precepts" (1999:62). This "middle path" is apparent in a number of studies surveying the social acceptability of abortion through self-administered questionnaires. These demonstrate that the Thai public is willing to allow abortion in certain circumstances not currently permitted by law, such as on the grounds of fetal deformity or mental illness of the mother (see the review in The Population Council 1981). Generally, elites are more liberal in their views and rural people more conservative. The Institute of Population Studies (1982) found that a majority of both rural and urban respondents approved of abortion in cases of mentally ill or disabled mothers who could not bring up a child, when the pregnancy was dangerous to maternal health, or if the woman had a hereditary disease that could affect the unborn child. Phuapradit et al. (1986) investigated attitudes among medical professionals, finding 69% favored a more liberalized abortion law and 17% favored complete legalization. The medical professionals expressed widespread approval for abortion in cases of rape, incest, threat to maternal health, mental illness and fetal abnormalities. More recently, Lerdmaleewong (1998) surveyed medical professionals in Bangkok, finding that the majority approved of abortion on the grounds of rape, women infected with HIV, and women infected with German measles. However, 70% of nursing and medical students would not support abortions on the grounds of economic disadvantage, large family size, student status, or low or high maternal age.

MOVEMENT FOR THE LIBERALIZATION
OF THE ABORTION LAW

Despite the evidence of widespread acceptance of a more liberal abortion law, so far all attempts to amend the law in Thailand have failed. Unlike many countries where the pro-choice movement draws from a broad grassroots constituency, in Thailand, advocacy to amend the abortion legislation has largely revolved around a handful of women's groups, concerned lawyers, prominent doctors, academics and journalists concentrated in Bangkok. Advocates of reform cannot draw upon a broad women's movement. In part this reflects the political culture of Thailand which until recently has provided little space for popular participation in policy and legislative reform. It also speaks to the continued ambivalence over the meanings of "feminism" and "rights" in Thailand. Opponents to reform draw upon religious opposition to abortion and argue that any amendments will lead to an acceptance of "free" abortion under any circumstance, less sexual responsibility, and an increase in the number of abortions. It should also be recognized that, as an illegal activity, abortion services are a lucrative business and it serves many people's interests to keep abortion illegal and expensive.

The abortion issue first arose in public debate in Thailand during the early 1970s, around the same time as the introduction of state family planning programs. A number of studies at this time began to document the extent of induced abortions and the substantial morbidity and mortality suffered by women. The closest Thailand ever got to reforming the law occurred in September 1981 when the House of Representatives passed an amendment to the abortion bill by 79 votes to 3. Three months later, in December 1981, the amended bill was rejected by the Senate by a vote of 147 to one, due to an intensive campaign against the bill by a coalition of concerned religious groups. This was spearheaded by Chamlong Srimuang, who was Vice-President of the Buddhist Association of Thailand and a devout member of the Buddhist Santi Asoke movement preaching a return to fundamental Buddhist lifestyles and values (see Whittaker 2001 for details). It was passed back to the House of Representatives but parliament was dissolved and no further action taken.

Repeated attempts to reintroduce the bill in February 1983 and again in April 1988 failed, again due to an emotional media campaign by Chamlong who was by then a Senator. By April 1990, when an amendment again passed for consideration, Chamlong had started the *Palang Tham* party and was an extremely popular politician. He once again took a stance against any amendment to the law. But while it was await-ing scheduling on the House agenda, the Chatichai government was ousted in a no-confidence vote.

A highly publicized raid on an abortion clinic in 1994 again stimu-lated wide public debate and resulted in a number of organizations, in-cluding the Ministry of Health, legal organizations, religious groups, academics and women's rights activists to debate the issue. The govern-ment opened "Daoprasuk Clinics" at public hospitals, to counsel women with unplanned pregnancies. Not surprisingly, these clinics proved un-popular. In the absence of any legal framework, they could not offer women any choice other than to continue their pregnancies.

In response to the growing AIDS epidemic, in February 1996, the Thai Medical Council lobbied parliament to make amendments to the Bill to allow abortions in the cases of pregnancies where the child might be born mentally retarded, or in the case of HIV positive mothers (*Bangkok Post* 9 February 1996; Khaykaew 1995). To date, however, such abortions remain technically illegal, although widespread. Some hospitals attempt to circumvent the legalities by citing mental health problems on the part of the mother as the reason for a legal termination, but remain on tenuous legal grounds. Anecdotal evidence from people working with people living with HIV/AIDS suggests that a number of women with HIV in rural areas who wish to terminate their pregnancies have had enormous difficulty in locating a doctor prepared to provide this service (Tansubhapol 1997). In October 1998 the Ministry of Jus-tice drafted a new law allowing women with HIV/AIDS to have legal terminations; however, recently the Council of State ruled out such grounds (*Bangkok Post* 7 November 2000). The Medical Council re-cently reported the formation of a panel to again consider the possibili-ties of legalizing abortion in the interests of the health of a mother (*Bangkok Post* 12 January 2001).

As noted above, groups such as the Foundation for Women, the net-work of academics known as the Thai Reproductive Health Advocacy Network, some members of the Thai Medical Council, some members working with the Ministry of Public Health, and legal groups continue to lobby to have the abortion laws revised. Actual legislative change however, is likely to be slow (Nataya Bunpakdi and Kanokwan Tharawan 2000). Along with abortion law reform, these groups stress the need for better counseling, the need for society to provide support and remove stigma from unmarried mothers, and better sex education for young people (Kitipong Kitayarak 1994; Withun U'ngprapan 1994). Consid-erable lobbying has continued in major government ministries and these groups are optimistic that the present parliament with the first fully elected Senate may provide the best prospect yet for change.

CONCLUSIONS

Abortion remains a highly contested issue in Thai society. The stories of women such as Nang Su and Nang Oi remind us that, despite the illegalities and the risks, abortion continues to be widely practiced in Thailand. As Germain notes, "laws do not stop abortion; they simply make it unsafe" (1989). Behind the debate and rhetoric live real women making difficult decisions. Within the restrictive legal context, risk is stratified along economic lines. Women's access to a safe abortion is determined by the amount of money they can mobilize. Women without access to money are often forced to resort to abortions through untrained practitioners. Even in private clinics with medically trained staff, women have no guarantees as to the quality of care they will receive. Their accounts speak eloquently of the power relations that directly impinge upon women's health.

In addition, this paper demonstrates the diversity of moral perspectives on abortion in Thailand. While not accepting the concept of the right to abortion on demand, the Thai public appears to be more tolerant of abortion under various circumstances than the present law reflects. While abortion is generally considered to be undesirable, there is an acknowledgement that, under some circumstances, women should be given access to safe abortions by trained staff. Although women such as Nang Su and Nang Oi may be aware of the illegality and believe that abortion constitutes a serious Buddhist sin, nevertheless, the economic and social realities of their lives are the salient factors in their decisions.

Finally, there is an ongoing campaign for abortion law reform in Thailand. Whilst falling short of advocating a woman's right to choose, it recognizes unsafe abortion as a major public health priority that needs to be addressed by the Thai government. The challenge remains to see the rhetoric of the policy debate made into reality.

NOTES

1. The definition of health in the legislation is ambiguous, but is generally interpreted to mean a woman's physical health.

2. These figures are based upon definitions under the International Classification of Disease (ICD) (Alpha Research 1997; Alpha Research Co. Ltd. and Manager Informa-

tion Services 1994). Between the 1992 and 1994 figures, the ICD underwent a revision and so the definitions may have been altered slightly.

3. The survey sample was predominated by married women (98% had ever been married and 92% were currently married) with an average age of 31 years.

4. Transliterations of words in Thai and the local Lao language follow a modified version of the Royal transliteration system. Tones and long vowels are not indicated in this system. Exceptions include place names, famous people's names and authors' names where the transcription follows that customarily used. Thai language references are listed alphabetically in the reference list under the first name of authors following Thai convention.

REFERENCES

Alpha Research. (1997). *Pocket Thailand Public Health 1997.* Bangkok: Alpha Research Co. Ltd.

Alpha Research and Manager Information Services. (1994). *Pocket Thailand Public Health 1995.* Bangkok: Alpha Research Co. Ltd., Manager Information Services.

Bleek, W. (1987). Lying Informants: A Fieldwork Experience from Ghana, *Population and Development Review* 13 (2), 314-321.

Boonthai, N. and S. Warakamin. (2001). Induced Abortion: A Nationwide Survey in Thailand. Paper presented at The XXV International Congress of the Medical Women's International Association (MWIA) on Women's Health in a Multicultural World, 19-23 April, Sydney.

Chaturachinda, K., S. Tangtrakul, S. Pongthai, W. Phuapradit, A. Phausopone, V. Benchakan, and J. J. Clinton. (1981). Abortion: An Epidemiologic Study at Ramathibodi Hospital, *Studies In Family Planning* 12 (6/7), 257-262.

Coeytaux, F., A. Leonard, and E. Royston. (1989). *Methodological Issues in Abortion Research. Proceedings of a seminar presented under the auspices of the Population Council's Robert H Ebert Program on Critical Issues in Reproductive Health, in collaboration with International Projects Assistance Services and the World Health Organization.* New York: The Population Council.

Germain, A. (1989). The Christopher Tietze International Symposium: An Overview, *International Journal of Gynecology and Obstetrics* Supplement 3, 1-8.

Hardacre, H. (1997). *Marketing the Menacing Fetus in Japan.* Berkeley and Los Angeles: University of California Press.

Helitzer-Allen, D., M. Makhambera, and A.M. Wangel. (1994). Obtaining Sensitive Information: The Need for More Than Focus Groups, *Reproductive Health Matters* 3 (May), 75-82.

Huntington, D., B. Mensch, and N. Toubia. (1993). A New Approach to Eliciting Information About Induced Abortion, *Studies in Family Planning* 24 (2), 120-124.

Institute of Population Studies. (1982). *Knowledge and Attitudes Concerning Abortion Practice in Urban and Rural Areas of Thailand.* Bangkok: Institute of Population Studies, Chulalongkorn University.

Kanokwan Tarawan. (2000) [2543]. *Rai gnan pon wijai bu'ang ton banteuk prasopkan khong phuying thi tung thong mu'a mai phrom* (Preliminary Research Findings: Recording the Experiences of Women with Unplanned Pregnancies). Paper presented at a seminar, *Thang lu 'ak khong phuying ti tung thong mu 'a mai phrom* (Choices for Woman with Unplanned Pregnancies), 6 July, Bangkok: Amari Watergate Hotel (In Thai).

Khaykaew, T. (1995). Thailand: Abortion Plea for AIDS Virus Women. *Bangkok Post*, 26 November.

Kitipong Kitayarak. (1994) [2537]. *Putcha-wisatchana:matrakan thang kotmai kap panha kan tham thang* (Question-Answer: Legal Standards and the Abortion Problem). Paper presented at the seminar *Matrakan thang kotmai kap panha kan tham thang* (Legislation and The Abortion Problem) (n.d.), Bangkok: Institute of Criminal Law, Office of Public Prosecution (In Thai).

Koetsawang, S. (1993). Illegally Induced Abortion in Thailand. Paper presented at the IPPF SEAO Regional Programme Advisory Panel Meeting on Abortion, 29-30 October 1993, Bali, Indonesia.

Koetsawang, S., Saha, A., and S. Pachauri. (1978). Study of "Spontaneous" Abortion in Thailand, *International Journal of Gynaecology and Obstetrics* 15 (4), 361-368.

Ladipo, O. A. (1989). Preventing and Managing Complications of Induced Abortion in Third World Countries, *International Journal of Gynecology and Obstetrics* Supplement 3, 21-28.

Lerdmaleewong, M., and C. Francis. (1998). Abortion in Thailand: A Feminist Perspective, *Journal of Buddhist Ethics*, 5.

Narkavonnakit, T., and T. Bennett. (1981). Health Consequences of Induced Abortion in Rural Northeast Thailand, *Studies in Family Planning* 12 (2), 58-65.

Nataya Bunpakdi, and Kanokwan Tharawan. (2000) [2543]. *Khabuankan khlu 'an wai phu 'a sitthi nai kan tham thang* (The Abortion Rights Movement), Paper presented at a seminar *Khabuan kan phuying kap kan mu 'ang ru 'ang rang kai satri* (The Process of Women and Woman's Bodies Politics), 6 March, Bangkok: SD Avenue Hotel (In Thai).

Phongpaichit, P., and C. Baker. (1995). *Thailand: Economy and Politics.* Kuala Lumpur: Oxford University Press.

Phuapradit, W., B. Sirivongs, and K. Chaturachinda. (1986). Abortion: An Attitude Study of Professional Staff at Ramathibodi Hospital, *Journal of The Medical Association of Thailand* 69 (1), 22-7.

Pinchun, P., and T. Chullapram. (1993). A 10-Year Review of Maternal Mortality in Chon Buri Hospital, Thailand, *Journal of The Medical Association of Thailand* 76 (6), 308-13.

Pongthai, S., W. Phuapradit, and K. Chaturachinda. (1984). Illegally Induced Abortion: Observation at Ramathibodi Hospital, *Journal of The Medical Association of Thailand* 67 (Supplement 2), 50-3.

Rabiabloke, C., and S. Wilairat. (1998). *Thailand National Family Planning Programme.* Nonthaburi: Family Planning and Population Division, Department of Health.

Ratanakul, P. (1999). Socio-Medical Aspects of Abortion in Thailand. In D. Keown. (ed.) *Buddhism and Abortion* (pp. 53-66). Honolulu: University of Hawaii Press.

Rattakul, P. (1971). Septic Abortion: The Scourge of Modern Obstetrics, *Journal of The Medical Association of Thailand* 54 (5), 312-319.

Rauyajin, O. (1979). *Induced Abortion: Facts and Prospect in Thailand.* Bangkok: Faculty of Social Sciences and Humanities, Mahidol University.

Tansubhapol, K. (1997). The Right to Choose. *Bangkok Post,* September 20, 1997.

Thailand, Ministry of Public Health. (1984) *Intensive Study of Rural Traditional Abortion in Thailand.* Bangkok: Ministry of Public Health, Special Projects Section, Family Health Division, Department of Health.

Thailand, Ministry of Public Health. (1990). *Wikrhaw comun satri kap sukhaphap. Data Analysis on Women and Health.* Bangkok: Thai Population Information Centre, Family Health Division, Department of Health, Ministry of Public Health.

Thailand, Ministry of Public Health. (1993). *Sathiti prachagon lae kan anamai khrop khrua lem 3. Selected Population and Family Health Statistics, 1992.* Bangkok: Thai Population Information Centre, Family Health Division, Department of Health, Ministry of Public Health.

The Population Council. (1981). *Abortion in Thailand: A Review of the Literature.* Bangkok: The Population Council.

Toongsuwan, S., C. Bhadrakom, and C. Usavajindawatn. (1973). Therapeutic Abortions in Siriraj Hospital, *Journal of the Medical Association of Thailand* 56 (4), 237-240.

Whittaker, A. (2000). *Intimate Knowledge: Women and Their Health in Northeast Thailand.* Sydney: Allen and Unwin.

Whittaker, A. (2001). Conceiving the Nation: Representations of Abortion in Thailand, *Asian Studies Review* 25 (4), 423-451.

Whittaker, A. (2002). 'The Truth of Our Day by Day Lives': Abortion Decision-Making in Rural Thailand, *Culture, Health and Sexuality* 4 (1), 1-20.

Withun U'ngprapan. (1994) [2537]. *Kotmai tham thang khor to yang ti yang mai yut (Abortion Law: The Unfinished Debate).* Bangkok: Gender Press (In Thai).

Index

T - #0588 - 101024 - C0 - 212/152/8 - PB - 9780789019899 - Gloss Lamination